Dr Atk
New
Diet
Cookbook

Dr Atkins
New
Diet
Cookbook

mouthwatering meals for one of the
world's most effective diets

By Dr Robert C. Atkins, with Fran Gare, m.s.

Vermilion
LONDON

We would like especially to acknowledge Nancy Mahoney, M.S., R.D., for her nutritional research on the recipes.

10

First published in the U.S. in 1994 by M. Evans & Company, Inc.
First published in the United Kingdom in 2003 by
Vermilion, an imprint of Ebury Press
Random House UK Ltd.
Random House
20 Vauxhall Bridge Road
London SW1V 2SA

Random House Australia (Pty) Limited
20 Alfred Street, Milsons Point, Sydney,
New South Wales 2061, Australia

Random House New Zealand Limited
18 Poland Road, Glenfield,
Auckland 10, New Zealand

Random House (Pty) Limited
Endulini, 5A Jubilee Road, Parktown 2193, South Africa

Random House UK Limited Reg. No. 954009
www.randomhouse.co.uk
Papers used by Vermilion are natural, recyclable products
made from wood grown in sustainable forests.

A CIP catalogue record is available for this book from the
British Library.

ISBN: 0091889464

Printed and bound in Great Britain by
Bookmarque Ltd, Croydon, Surrey

Contents

Chapter 1
Introduction   1

Chapter 2
Four Diets in One   9

Chapter 3
Meal Plans   20
    The Induction Diet   20
    The Ongoing Weight-Loss Diet   25
    The Premaintenance Diet   30
    The Yeast-Free Diet   35
    The Maintenance Diet   41
    The Yeast-Free Maintenance Diet   42

Chapter 4
Recipes   43
    Eggs   44
    Appetizers   58
    Soups   69
    Salads   79
    Salad Dressings   92
    Meat   100
    Poultry   124
    Fish and Shellfish   140
    Pasta   156
    Bread   161

Vegetables   164
Sauces   180
Desserts   189
Beverages   217

Appendices   224
    Special Menus for Entertaining   225
    Nutritional Supplementation   229
    Carbohydrate Gram Counter   232

Index   241

1 | *Introduction*

You have all seen diet cookbooks, but for the past 20 years I suspect you haven't seen one like this. This isn't a copycat cookbook. It doesn't attempt to refurbish and bring to life the tired and repetitious diet styles of the recent past. In fact, if you start leafing through the recipes, you'll be in for the shock of your life. *Where's the diet?* you'll say. What happened to the austerity? No austerity, no diet, right? *Wrong!*

What sort of diet is this, then? Just glance at the wonderful, mouth-watering recipes Fran Gare has prepared for this book. Yes, they appear non-dietetic because they're *not* fat-restricted. You quickly notice that oil, butter, and mayonnaise appear in them. *Why, Dr. Atkins, this is not the food of weight loss!* You tremble. Don't! This is the food of weight loss, and you can become slim eating it. (And, better yet, healthy.) But, I have to tell you that if you're relying on fat restriction to get you slim, this cookbook is certainly not for you.

On the other hand, if, like so many of the people I meet, you've been trying fat restriction and getting nowhere, I'll hazard a guess that this cookbook and the diet principles that go with it are exactly what you need.

You need a new start; new principles; a diet that works.

The success I promise is not done by magic. Low-carbohydrate dieting is the answer, and that means the application of well-attested facts about overweight that you've probably never heard about. Quite simply, since the late 1970s a simplistic theory of weight loss that focuses obsessively on dietary fat and by implication teaches the old, stale doctrine that gaining or losing weight is just a matter of calorie consumption has ruled the roost.

To know how simplistic it is to look at overweight that way, you only have to consider the different people you know, their different body types, and their different levels of appetite. Right away you'll see that there's no necessary connection between how much you eat and how heavy you are or between eating a lot of fat and being fat. You've surely noticed that folks who eat bacon and eggs for breakfast aren't consistently overweight. Nor folks who eat steaks or butter. Yet the restriction of fat has become the basis of a whole new weight-loss industry. Weight Watchers and its many imitators wage the battle of the bulge. Low-fat tips crowd the pages of women's magazines, and dire warnings resound from medical authorities on high.

And, as a result, we as a nation are without question and by all statistical measures eating less fat. The American public must be getting slimmer. Is it? That's a question I can easily answer. NHANES, the major government survey that tracks the weight patterns of the nation, found just last year that from 1980 to 1990, the percentage of overweight American adults went up from 26 percent of the population to 34 percent—a truly massive and astonishing 30 percent jump. If pudge-proneness is a virus, then tens of millions of us caught it even as we struggled to obey our antifat mentors.

Food for thought here. I know I haven't shocked you enough, so let me talk about eating. After all, this is a book that promises to be a source of the richest and most diverse dining pleasure. Disguise it though they may, most diet cookbook authors want to teach you how you can like carrot sticks and granola, skim milk and skinless chicken, celery sticks and butterless toast. They set a hard task for themselves. In their attempt to deploy a few delicious salads (though no more delicious than the ones our own Fran Gare will reveal to you), they are fundamentally working from poverty. Good cuisine has always rooted itself firmly in luxurious fat. That's why I feel confident you're going to relate to a diet and a cookbook that allows you New England Clam Chowder and Spicy Spare Ribs, Steak Au Poivre, Pâté and Roast Chicken, Duck in Red Wine, and desserts like Cheesecake and Chocolate Ice Cream.

I can see your mouth has fallen open, partly from appetite and partly from disbelief. *Dr. Atkins,* you're saying, *I heard you mention the merits of low carbohydrate dieting and I was perfectly willing to suspend my disbelief, but this is beyond the beyond. I've been reading magazine articles for the past dozen years trying to wean me from these delights. You're not serious!*

COULDN'T BE MORE SERIOUS, MY FRIEND

So, what gives? I'll tell you frankly out of my experience in advising overweight patients for a quarter of a century. In spite of all the hoopla and hysteria of the preceding years, most overweight men and women are *not* particularly sensitive to dietary fat.

What makes them fat and keeps them fat is a disorder of their *carbohydrate* metabolism. The foods they can't handle are *carbohydrate* foods. Trying to lose weight by fat restriction is torture for them because it doesn't address the *carbohydrate* basis of their problem.

Many of our major health problems and most of our weight problems are indeed nutritional, but they spring from eating the refined, processed, and devitalized food of the modern world, not from eating too many steaks or chicken breasts. I'd like to assure you that the health-problem foods that are really waiting to ambush you are sugar and sweeteners, hydrogenated oils and white flour, margarine and fizzy drinks.

Do you realize that if you're overweight, there's a better than 90 percent chance that you have a problem with blood sugar and insulin levels? There's a very good chance that you are or will become diabetic. You're putting yourself at risk for heart disease. You probably suffer from fatigue and irritability that's totally curable if you eat a low-carbohydrate diet. And there's sound scientific evidence for what I'm telling you now that is largely being ignored.

I'd like to see you on the Atkins diet not just because it will slim you down remarkably, not just because it's delightful to imagine eating the delicious recipes Fran has prepared for you, but because you deserve to be a healthy person. The Atkins diet is a diet that reverses hypertension, controls diabetes, ends fatigue, corrects many eating and digestive disorders, and greatly reduces allergies.

Low-carbohydrate diets have often gotten a bum rap in the press and for that reason I hope that before you go on the Atkins diet you'll begin by having blood tests and measuring your blood pressure. After you've been on the diet for a few weeks, have these numbers checked again. Then, if your family or friends criticize you for doing something so unorthodox as ignoring the low-fat dogmas prevalent now, you'll be able to point to the irrefutable, numerical improvements in such health indicators as cholesterol and triglyceride levels and blood pressure. There's nothing like showing people that you're getting healthy even while they're watching you get slim.

INSULIN, OVERWEIGHT, AND YOU

If—as is most likely—you're among the overweight to whom my description of carbohydrate sensitivity applies, then your weight problem is caused by a problem with insulin, the hormone produced in the pancreas that we cannot live without. This is a scientific fact never mentioned in the weight-loss manuals of the antifat brigades.

Yet obesity is almost always found together with an excessive release of insulin after eating, the medical term for which is hyperinsulinism. When you eat, your body produces blood sugar (glucose). If you eat carbohydrate food, especially the refined carbohydrates I mentioned above, the glucose level goes up rapidly. Insulin is released to lower it. The insulin enables some of that glucose to be used for energy and stores the rest as . . . fat.

In fact, one wise scientist referred to insulin as "the fat-producing hormone."

Now if you want to lose weight, I've just told you the secret. Simply restrict the foods that stimulate excessive insulin release. Carbohydrates provide that kind of stimulation. Fats and proteins don't.

You simply need to severely restrict your consumption of carbohydrates (down to one or two small salads a day to start with), and you're on a weight-loss plan that has an unparalleled record of success.

And success doesn't stop when the pounds are off. I know you don't just want to lose weight, you want to keep it off.

Weight regain is the demon that bedevils dieters. They put time and effort and high hopes into adhering to a diet, and they lose 10 or 14 kilos, or perhaps 25 or 30 kilos, and then, presto, six months or eight months or a year after the diet is done they're back up where they were before. It's almost worse than never having lost.

No need for that on this diet plan. The Atkins maintenance diet is a natural transition from the initial weight-loss diet, and on it the vast majority of my dieters maintain their slimness. The lifetime diet you can move into once you're at your ideal weight is a healthy omnivorous diet that includes meats, fish, fowl, vegetables, nuts, seeds, grains, and fruits and starches in moderation.

THIS IS WHAT YOU CAN EXPECT

Let me mention just a few things—besides good food—that you can expect to experience on the Atkins diet. Those of you who want to do the diet would be well advised to obtain *Dr. Atkins' New Diet Revolution* and learn step-by-step the essentials of successful low-carbohydrate dieting. I know many of you already have and now you're turning to this cookbook to make your diet experience more enjoyable. For those of you who are newcomers to the Atkins diet, this chapter aims to make it possible for you to begin the diet and carry it through with success. The final pages of this chapter will explain the four stages of the Atkins lifetime-diet plan.

By following the simple rules, you'll find yourself on a weight-loss program that has the following surprising characteristics. Study them carefully for very few diets can claim even one of them.

This is a diet that:

- Sets no limit on the amount of food you can eat.
- Completely excludes hunger from the dieting experience.
- Includes rich and luxurious foods that you've never associated with dieting before.
- Reduces your appetite by a perfectly natural function of the body.
- Gives you a metabolic edge so significant that the whole concept of watching calories will become absurd to you.
- Produces steady weight loss, even if you have experienced dramatic failures on other diets.
- Is so perfectly adapted to use as a lifetime diet that, unlike most diets, the lost weight won't come back.
- Consistently produced improvements in most of the health problems that accompany overweight.

I'm sure you wonder how all this is possible. Why does the diet work? How will my appetite be reduced? What's all this talk of a metabolic edge? Those were all the questions I hoped you'd ask. Listen.

KETOSIS/LIPOLYSIS

On the Atkins diet, you'll lose weight without hunger. To most dieters that's the miraculous part. No more counting calories, skimping on portions, rising from the table with an ache of appetite still present and unaccounted for. I not only tell my dieters, *Well, if you're hungry, eat!* but I take pleasure in the fact that low-carbohydrate dieting suppresses appetite. Most of you will find that the change in your appetite level is one of the most astonishing experiences of your dieting life.

You see, your body was designed to suppress hunger during

periods of food deprivation. If any of you have fasted or watched other people fast, you'll have noticed that after the first two days hunger disappears. Carbohydrate restriction produces the same phenomenon.

What does the body of a faster or a low-carbohydrate dieter do to provide energy? It burns off its own stored fat. In the case of a fast you'll also burn off muscle tissue, which is not advisable and can even be dangerous. On a low-carbohydrate diet, you burn off *nothing but fat*.

In the metabolic pecking order, the first fuel that the body uses for energy—glucose—is derived from carbohydrate food. But when you drastically restrict carbohydrate intake, very little glucose is produced in your bloodstream after you've eaten. Your crafty metabolism appraises the alternatives and for two days after the diet begins it turns to stored carbohydrate (called glycogen) to power its operations. Once that is gone, your body moves down the pecking order. It turns to its own fat for fuel. Presto! you've begun to lose weight.

You enter a state called ketosis because among the by-products of fat burning are compounds called ketone bodies. They're your new-found source of energy. Be assured, your body is just as happy using them as it was using glucose. Another name for the whole process is lipolysis, which means "the dissolving of fat."

As you go into ketosis/lipolysis, the appetite suppression I just mentioned occurs. Because this usually results in a decrease in your intake of calories, your rate of weight loss is accelerated. But if you continue to eat as many calories as you did before the diet started, you will generally lose weight anyway only at a slower pace.

YOUR METABOLIC ADVANTAGE
This "extra" weight loss is the result of a very exciting side benefit of low-carbohydrate dieting called a metabolic advantage. Very simply—and this has been repeatedly demonstrated in scientific studies—*a person who's eating a strict low-carbohydrate diet loses more weight at whatever his or her level of caloric intake is than he or she would be losing if eating the same number of calories on any other type of diet.* Startling, but at least ten studies conducted in the '60s, '70s, and '80s demonstrated that effect. A low-carbohydrate diet is a calorically wasteful diet. More calories are burned off by your metabolism than on any other diet.

I'm sure I don't need to tell you what an advantage this is. You don't need to concentrate on restricting calories; all you need to do is keep your intake of carbohydrate at such a level that you're in ketosis and enjoying the metabolic advantage nature has provided for you. From that there automatically follows appetite suppression and accelerated rate of weight loss per unit of caloric intake.

Let me emphasize one simple fact: Your body *wants* you to use up your fat stores. It elaborates all sorts of messenger chemicals to facilitate the burning of your stored fat—they're called fat mobilizers. The fat mobilizers redirect your metabolic processes so that you comfortably switch from your normal sugar-burning pathway to the alternative pathway where fat is your body's—and your brain's—primary fuel.

Ketosis/lipolysis is the happiest condition a dieter can be in. Not only does it work, but it requires no willpower, no hunger, and no suffering of any kind. After two or three days of adjustment to the diet, most of you will feel better and more energetic than you've felt in years.

Being on the Atkins diet is a great convincer, but you have to bring some degree of resolution and commitment to your nutritional changeover. A halfhearted low-carbohydrate diet may make you feel physically better, but it probably won't produce much weight loss. Smooth, consistent weight loss is a consequence of so severely restricting carbohydrate intake that you do go into ketosis and begin to burn your own fat for fuel.

To do this you must initally cut down your carbohydrates to one or two small salads or a salad and a helping of vegetables per day. Bread, pasta, sugar, and starchy foods in general will not be allowed while you're in the weight-loss phase of your diet plan. Once you've reached your ideal weight you'll be able to cautiously increase your intake of carbohydrate foods.

OTHER ESSENTIALS OF THE ATKINS DIET

Knowing whether you're in ketosis/lipolysis or not is obviously crucial to your success. Some people play it by ear (or ounce). If they're losing weight they know they're following the game plan. I think it's more effective to get Bioketone testing strips, which you can put in your urine once a day (preferably in the evening). If the strips turn purple, you know you're in ketosis.

Another crucial aspect of dietary success is nutritional supplementation. In the strict early phase of the diet, which I call the Induction phase, you'll need vitamins and minerals to keep you at a healthy level for all nutrients. Even when you're at the advanced and more liberalized levels of the diet I strongly advise supplementation because it's good for you. See "Nutritional Supplementation" in the appendices for a description of what your basic multivitamin formula should include.

BE PREPARED

My other advice for the beginning Atkins dieter is in the area of preparation. Prepare your relatives and prepare your kitchen. Qualitatively speaking, this is a strict diet. There's no room for cheating. I can already hear your spouse saying, "Just this one little piece of cake won't hurt you." It will. You can't do the diet that way.

So start by telling the folks you live with just what you intend to do. Tell them that you take your diet seriously, and you'd appreciate their doing the same. If they question the wisdom of a high-protein diet that isn't interested in fat restriction, tell them to watch and wait. When they see how terrific you feel and how good you look, their temptation to criticize will start to fade away. Be diplomatic and gentle but firm. Eating is a very emotional habit, and changes in the way you eat affect everyone around you. Nonetheless, this is your diet, not your relatives'.

As for your kitchen, if you live alone it will be easy. Invite some friends over to finish off the ice cream, and give all your forbidden foods away to friends and neighbours. If there are others in the house, and they're not going to be on this diet, then simply see that there are separate portions of such forbidden foods as bread, potatoes, and sugar-laden desserts for them. The main course, the salads, and the vegetables will be suitable for everyone.

Now, before you turn to the wonderful part of this book (the food!), look at the next chapter and make sure you know how you'll do the series of diets that together comprise the Atkins diet. This is going to be your gateway to a lifetime of eating pleasure and dieting success.

2 | *Four Diets in One*

This chapter is designed for those of you who haven't read *Dr. Atkins' New Diet Revolution*. It will give, I hope, a simple and effective description of the Atkins diet in its four stages.

These are:

1. The Induction Diet
2. The Ongoing Weight-Loss Diet
3. The Premaintenance Diet
4. The Maintenance Diet

These four stages are an effective way of breaking up and explaining what—for you—will be one continuous lifetime diet. The Induction diet gets you into weight loss with a bang; the Ongoing Weight-Loss diet carries you through the weeks or months of weight loss needed to get you close to your ideal weight; the Premaintenance diet takes you the final few steps and eases your transition to what is perhaps the most important diet of all; and that is the Maintenance diet—your lifetime ticket to health and slimness. Let's take them in order.

GETTING STARTED

The Induction diet—your start-up diet—is very strict in its limitation of carbohydrates. *Because of its rigor, this phase of the diet is not appropriate for pregnant women and people with severe kidney disease.* You'll only be eating 15 to 20 grams of carbohydrates on it, which might be two medium salads and a helping of vegetables. The purpose of this strictness is to ensure that your body does indeed go into ketosis/lipolysis, does begin releasing fat-mobilizing hormones that will suppress your appetite, and does, after the first two or three days, begin to consume your own fat. This is what you're working toward initially, and your success is pretty well assured.

Once you're in ketosis, your body has made a transition from burning carbohydrate (glucose) for fuel to employing its alternative metabolic pathway that was evolved millions of years ago to enable you to survive periods of famine. You now break down fat, and the by-products of this fat breakdown—ketone bodies—are consumed for energy.

This is the basic Atkins diet, so let me explain it in full. The other three diets are careful, gradual liberalizations of the Induction diet, and they'll be easy to explain once you're grounded in the Induction diet.

THE RULES OF THE INDUCTION DIET

1. *Your diet must contain no more than 20 grams of carbohydrates a day.* For most people, induction of ketosis/lipolysis can be achieved on this intake. This allows for approximately 180 g of salad vegetables (loosely packed) or 120 g of salad plus about 150 g of cooked vegetables in the below 10 percent carbohydrate category.
2. You are no longer on a quantitative diet. Therefore you should adjust the quantities to your appetite. When hungry, eat the amount that makes you feel satisfied but not stuffed. When not hungry, eat nothing or just a small protein snack to accompany your vitamins.
3. You are, however, on a qualitative diet. This means that if the food is not on your diet, you are to have absolutely none of it. Your "just this one taste won't hurt" rationalization is the kiss of death on this diet. Addicts will find this rule builds character in a hurry.
4. Your diet will consist of pure proteins (not many of those in nature, however), pure fats (this means butter, olive oil, and mayonnaise are permitted), and combinations of protein and fat (this is the mainstay of your diet). Foods that are protein-and-carbohydrate or fat-and-carbohydrate are *not* on this diet, because carbohydrate is not on this diet.
5. Using a carbohydrate gram counter, one could find other combinations totaling less than 20 grams of carbohydrate. One would be using foods like nuts, seeds, olives, avocados,

cheeses, cream and soured cream, lemon and lime juices, and low-carbohydrate diet foods. Don't assume these foods are low, unless you absolutely know the carbohydrate content of the portion you are eating. In the Carbohydrate Gram Counter on page 232, I will include the carbohydrate content in grams of the foods you may include on this 14-day *Induction* diet as well as on more liberal levels of the diet that you will be doing as your lifetime diet plan.

FREE FOODS:

MEAT	FISH	FOWL
Beef	Tuna	Chicken
Pork	Salmon	Turkey
Lamb	Sole	Duck
Bacon	Trout	Goose
Veal	Flounder	Guinea fowl
Ham	Sardines	Quail
Venison	Herring	Pheasant
in fact, all meat	*in fact, all fish*	*in fact, all fowl*

SHELLFISH	EGGS	CHEESE
Oysters	Scrambled	Matured and fresh
Mussels	Fried	Cow and goat
Clams	Poached	Cream cheese
Squid	Soft Boiled	Cottage cheese
Prawns	Hard Boiled	Swiss
Lobster	Devilled	Cheddar
Crab meat	Omelettes	Mozzarella
in fact, all shellfish	*in fact, all eggs*	*in fact, almost* all cheeses*

Exceptions: 1) delicatessen meats with nitrates or sugar added
2) products that are not exclusively meat, fish, or fowl, such as imitation fish

---

*All cheeses have some carbohydrate content, and quantities are governed by that. (See Carbohydrate Gram Counter.) No diet cheese, cheese spreads, or whey cheeses. Those with a known yeast infection, dairy allergy, or cheese intolerance must avoid cheese. Imitation cheese products are not allowed, except for Tofu (soy cheese)—but check carbohydrate content.

OTHER INDUCTION DIET FOODS:

Vegetables of 10 Percent Carbohydrate or Less

SALAD VEGETABLES:

Alfalfa Sprouts	Jicama	Parsley
Celery	Lamb's Lettuce	Peppers
Chicory	Lettuce	Radicchio
Chives	Mache	Radishes
Cucumber	Morels	Rocket
Endive	Mushrooms	Romaine (Cos)
Escarole	Olives	Sorrel
Fennel	Pak Choy	

SALAD HERBS:

Basil	Dill	Rosemary
Coriander	Oregano	Thyme

For salad dressing use the desired oil plus vinegar or lemon juice and spices. Grated cheese, chopped eggs, bacon, or fried pork rinds may be added.

VEGETABLES IN ADDITION TO SALAD VEGETABLES:

Artichoke Hearts	Chard	Pumpkin
Asparagus	Christophene	Rhubarb
Aubergine	Collard Greens	Sauerkraut
Avocado	Courgette	Spaghetti Squash
Bamboo Shoots	Dandelion Greens	Spinach
Bean Sprouts	Hearts of Palm	Spring Onions
Beet Greens	Kale	Stringless Beans
Broccoli	Kohlrabi	Summer Squash
Brussels Sprouts	Leeks	Tomato
Cabbage	Mangetout	Turnips
Cauliflower	Okra	Water Chestnuts
Celery Root (celeriac)	Onion	

SALAD GARNISHES:

Anchovies	Chopped Hard-Boiled Egg Yolk
Crumbled Crispy Bacon	Chopped Sautéed Mushrooms
Grated Cheese	Soured Cream

SPICES:

All spices to taste, but make sure sugar is not in the seasoning.

BEVERAGES:

Water
Mineral Water
Essence Flavoured Seltzer
 (must say "No Calories")
Decaffeinated coffee or tea
Diet Soda (read label)
Iced tea with artificial sweetener
Cream (double, single or
 whipping, or crème fraîche)
Natural and artificial orange
 drinks have some
 carbohydrate—they may be
 one of your options for a few
 grams

Spring Water
Club Soda
Herb Tea
 (no barley, dates, figs, sugar)
Caffeine is not allowed
Carbohydrate-free, artificially
 sweetened powder for making
 fruit-flavoured drinks
Clear consommé/bouillon (not
 all brands)
Grain Beverages (i.e., imitation
 coffee substitutes) are not
 allowed

FATS AND OILS:

Many fats, especially certain oils, are essential to good nutrition. Include a source of GLA (gamma-linolenic acid) and omega-3 oils (EPA, salmon oil, linseed oil). Olive oil (monounsaturated) is valuable. All vegetable oils are allowed. The best are canola, walnut, soybean, sesame, sunflower, and safflower oils, especially if they are labeled "cold pressed." Butter is allowed; margarine is not. Margarine should be avoided not because of its carbohydrate content but because it is a potential health hazard. Mayonnaise is permitted unless you are on a yeast restriction. The fat that is part of the meat or fowl you eat is permitted.

Avoid the seeming paradox provided by today's "diet foods." Understand why cream is allowed but not skim milk, why soured cream can be used but not yoghurt, why low-fat chicken breading is not allowed even though chicken may be pan-fried. The answer common to all of these seeming inconsistencies lies in the higher carbohydrate content of the low-fat dieter's foods.

ARTIFICIAL SWEETENERS:

Dieters must determine which artificial sweeteners agree with them, but the following are allowed: saccharine, aspartame, acesulfame-K.

Sweeteners such as sorbitol, mannitol, and other hexitols are not allowed, nor are any natural sweeteners ending in the letters -ose, such as maltose, fructose, and so on.

COMMON MISTAKES TO AVOID:

1. Note that the 14-day diet contains no fruit, bread, grains, starchy vegetables, dairy products other than cheese, cream, or butter.
2. Avoid diet products unless they specifically state "no carbohydrates." Most dietetic foods are for fat-restricted, not carbohydrate-restricted, diets.
3. The word sugarless is not sufficient. The product must state the carbohydrate content, and that's what you go by.
4. Many products you do not normally think of as foods such as chewing gum, cough syrups, and cough drops are filled with sugar and other caloric sweeteners and must be avoided.

THE ONGOING WEIGHT-LOSS DIET

You won't need to do the Induction diet for more than a couple of weeks. By that time, I feel confident that you'll not only be losing weight but feeling healthier than you have in years. Most people feel energized by a low-carbohydrate diet. On the weight-loss front, most of you will have seen five to ten pounds disappear, and that means you can now liberalize your intake of carbohydrate slightly. You've begun the Ongoing Weight-Loss diet, which will carry you pleasantly along for as many weeks or months as it takes to get you very close to your ideal weight.

This minor liberalization of carbohydrate is, of course, not an invitation to go back to eating the way you did before. What, in fact, you'll be doing is increasing the daily amount of carbohydrate by 5 grams at a time. You'll do this very gradually because you don't want to fall out of ketosis/lipolysis. I suggest that each week you increase your daily carbohydrate consumption by 5 grams. Typical 5-gram increments are 10 Brazil nuts or 20 macadamias, or half of an avocado or half a tomato, or 90 g of plain, unflavoured yoghurt, or 80g green beans or broccoli or $2^{1}/_{2}$ wafers of GG Bran Crispbread.

Those of you who have been chafing at the absolute restriction of alcohol on the induction diet might now add 125 ml of dry wine or 185 ml of a light beer, or 30 ml of whiskey or gin daily.

Yeast Infections

I have to tell you a little bit about yeast infections because—if you have them—they could derail your diet and blight your predestined success.

In my experience, more than a quarter of the patients I see have an overgrowth of one particular yeast, which is known as *Candida albicans*. *Candida* is a normal part of your body, one of four hundred species of bacteria resident in the human intestinal tract. In healthy competition with your other intestinal flora, *Candida* serves you well performing yeasty bacterial mission in your gut. But when some disturbance upsets the bacterial equilibrium in your body, a yeast infection can ensue. *Candida* overgrows, suppresses less aggressive bacteria, and causes a multitude of symptoms.

A short list of the problems a yeast infection can cause include lethargy; fatigue; depression; inability to concentrate; headaches; gastrointestinal disorders, including constipation, abdominal pain, gas, diarrhea, and bloating; respiratory ailments; and disorders of the urinary tract and reproductive organs. The most specific symptom is bloating—gas in the lower abdomen.

Let me repeat: A *Candida albicans* yeast infection will also make it very difficult to lose weight.

The four most common contributing causes to a yeast infection are:

1. A diet high in sugar and refined carbohydrates.
2. Antibiotics (more than 20 weeks in a lifetime would make *Candida* overgrowth a probability).
3. The mercury in silver dental fillings.
4. Birth control pills, prednisone, and other steroids.

This is an embarrassing list for medicine since the last three provokers of yeast overgrowth are all related to medical care. Perhaps that explains why *Candida* hasn't received nearly the attention it deserves.

If you think you have a yeast infection, you may need to see a physician who's experienced in treating them. In *Dr. Atkins' New Diet Revolution* I devote a chapter to *Candida* and its treatments. For now, let me simply say that whatever therapies your doctor proposes, he will certainly also tell you that you need to make alterations in the way you eat. Fermented and yeast-containing foods are inappropriate for a person who's suffering from yeast overgrowth. Please turn to the section on the yeast-free diet for further information on this dietary problem.

Of course, as you increase your carbohydrate consumption, you will see a gradual decrease in your rate of weight loss. That's fine. The purpose of this diet is not to lose weight in a hurry, but to get it off and *keep it off.* By slowing down your rate of loss, you go gradually toward your ultimate diet.

THE PREMAINTENANCE DIET

The Premaintenance diet is a further extension of the diet liberalisation that you went toward on the Ongoing Weight-Loss diet. When you're getting fairly close to your ultimate goal weight, it's very important that you lose weight slowly. Many of you are such determined dieters that this will be psychologically burdensome. You've got that final two or three kilos to go, you know you can do it in two weeks, why postpone success? Sorry, folks, that's not the best way to proceed. I think you should carve off those final pounds over the course of two or three months. Here's why.

The biggest problem with weight control is not the losing but the maintenance. How many celebrity dieters have you heard of who lost their weight in a crash program and then gained it back faster than they lost it? What you should do is just the opposite. Lose those final pounds with excruciating slowness so that by the time you say, "I'm there!" you'll be virtually eating your lifetime diet.

As for doing Premaintenance, it's simple. Either add another 10 grams of carbohydrate a day to what you've been eating on Ongoing Weight-Loss, or give yourself a 20-gram carbohydrate treat two or three times a week. You can even touch some forbidden starches. A bagel, a baked potato, some French toast, a slice of pizza, a side dish of lasagna. Or else add some of your favorite fruits—apples, oranges, grapefruits, peaches, bananas. As long as you don't start gaining weight but continue to lose at an almost imperceptible rate, you're doing fine.

GOING ON YOUR LIFETIME MAINTENANCE DIET

Now that you've arrived, offer yourself some well-deserved self-congratulation, and prepare for a slim lifetime.

As you already know, there's no shortage of delicious food for you to eat. The one scientific fact of importance that you must be aware of, however, is that once you've totally stopped your weight loss, your appetite will increase toward its normal level. For this reason, your lifetime maintenance diet will still be fairly restrictive of carbohydrate foods.

You'll need to find your own level, and that level will be what I call your Critical Carbohydrate Level for Maintenance. This is the level *above* which you *gain* weight. At this level, you will have enough carbohydrate restriction to keep *some* curbing of your appetite, and, for most of you, this will range between 40 and 90 grams of carbohydrate a day. Still considerably less than the average American consumption of 300 grams a day!

Here are my final suggestions for you happy dieters who have now reached your ideal weight.

1. Be food aware—meat, fish, fowl, nuts, seeds, vegetables, and occasional fruits and starches are the foods nature designed you to eat. Avoid processed foods. Eat fresh and natural to the best of your ability.
2. Avoid sugar and corn syrup and white flour and cornstarch like the plague. For most people these are the foods of overweight and ill health.
3. Individualize your diet. Try new foods. Create the diet that's right for you.
4. Consider the program of vitamin and mineral supplementation that's explained in Appendix 1 and that you've been using while you were on the weight-loss portion of the diet.
5. Use caffeine and alcohol in moderation.
6. If you regain more than 2.5 kilos of weight go right back to the Induction diet. Within two weeks you should find yourself back at your ideal weight.
7. Please do exercise. Though there isn't time to talk about it here, it's wonderful for health and very helpful in maintaining slimness.

Now for a final word about eating. . . .

ARE YOU READY TO BE HAPPY?

I can't guarantee that I'll make you wealthy and wise, but I have every intention of making you happy in your body. That doesn't just mean slim, it also means healthy and thrilled by the food you eat. It's simply essential that your foods thrill you. If they don't, how can I fulfill my promise that for you the Atkins diet will be a lifetime diet?

I want your new meals to provide you with every bit as much emotional satisfaction and eating happiness as your normal pre-Atkins way of eating did. Hopefully more. If we succeed at this, then there will be no reason for you to return to your old way of eating—the way that didn't work.

If you follow the suggestions that that ever-so-talented food wizard, Fran Gare, has prepared for you in this book, you will probably end up much better at cooking than you were before. This is no small advantage. Add to that the fact that on the Atkins maintenance diet, you will be eating sufficient fat to produce satiety and avoid disruptive blood sugar patterns, and I think you're an odds-on favorite to succeed.

Let me give you a dieting tip. One of the advantages of fat in your diet is that it buffers your changing blood sugar levels, it prevents swift, disturbing changes, and it thereby suppresses the craving for sweets. The successful effort to lower the amount of fat in the American diet over the past two decades has been bought at a crippling price. During this same period the American consumption of sugar has increased by 9 kilos yearly. That's not only a catastrophe for dieters but a catastrophe for health.

You may have heard of the French paradox. The French consume more fat than Americans (including four times as much butter and twice as much cheese), but they have less than half our heart attack rate. How can this be? It demands an answer, and the theorists of low fat have done a spectacularly ineffectual job of providing one. But the true answer is evident. We eat three times as much sugar as the French, and the research linking sugar to excess insulin production to heart disease is strong and growing stronger.

So don't be afraid of fat. Not only can you use it for weight loss, you can eat it in good health. The Atkins diet is not a high-fat diet since many of the junk food sources of fat are not permitted on it, but it is a diet that's unafraid of fat. The lifetime maintenance diet that will keep you slim is natural for human beings and well suited to the improvement of your health.

As you succeed on the Atkins diet and eat the scrumptious recipes Fran Gare has prepared for you, there will be one final question you'll have to ask yourself: Am I happier eating this way than I was before? Personally, I think nothing compares with smelling a delectable main course sizzling in the frying pan and experiencing appetite combined with the sure and certain knowledge that appetite is shortly to be gratified.

On many other diets people are asked, "Are you satisfied with the food?" and often they'll reply, "Oh, yes, I'm satisfied." All too often, these responses fail the acid test of dieting: The hopeful dieters who made them end up gaining their weight back and resuming their former eating patterns.

But so seldom does that happen with the diet you're committed to trying now. So very seldom. And, of course, that's because dieters are happier eating the Atkins way. Most of them feel better than they've felt in years, all of them look better, and, far from feeling deprived, they're luxuriating in a whole new world of delicious foods.

And now that I've said the magic words, *delicious foods,* please proceed to the rest of the book. I leave you in the capable hands of Fran Gare.

3 | *Meal Plans*

The Induction Diet

DAY 1

Breakfast

2–3 Eggs, *Poached, *Hard- or Soft-Boiled
4 rashers nitrate-free bacon
30g Cheddar cheese
Tea or decaffeinated coffee with 15 ml cream and sugar substitute

Lunch

*Chicken Salad Ham Rolls
*Orange Cooler

Dinner

*Spicy Cocktail
*Luscious Lamb
Tossed green salad with *Vinaigrette Cream Dressing

Snack

Cheese cubes

---

*Those dishes noted with an asterisk are found in Chapter 4, Recipes.

DAY 2

Breakfast

*Scrambled or *Sunny-Side Up and Over Easy eggs
2 slices smoked ham wrapped around a celery stick stuffed with 1 tablespoon of soft (cream) cheese
Tea or decaffeinated coffee with 15 ml cream and sugar substitute

Lunch

*¡Ole! Burger
½ cucumber, sliced, sprinkled with cayenne pepper

Dinner

*Salami and Parmesan
*Sole with Soured Cream
Tossed green salad with *Lime Dill Dressing
Tea or decaffeinated coffee with 15 ml cream and sugar substitute

Snack

*Hot Mint Chocolate Nog

DAY 3

Breakfast

>   *Cheese-Baked Eggs
>   2 sausage patties
>   Tea or decaffeinated coffee with 15 ml cream and sugar substitute

Lunch

>   *Chicken Croquettes on a bed of lettuce
>   *Orange Cooler

Dinner

>   *Soured Cream Clam Dip with fried pork rinds
>   *Fennel Red Snapper
>   Tossed green salad with *Dressing of the House
>   Tea or decaffeinated coffee with 15 ml cream and sugar substitute

Snack

>   *Vanilla Ice Cream

DAY 4

Breakfast

>   *Mocha Drink
>   *Herb Omelette

Lunch

>   *Sardine snack on lettuce leaves
>   Sliced celery and olives
>   Tea or decaffeinated coffee with 15 ml cream and sugar substitute

Dinner

>   *Tomato Lemon Aspic
>   *Lemon-Basted Roast Chicken
>   *Ricotta Sauce for Chicken
>   Tea or decaffeinated coffee with 15 ml cream and sugar substitute

Snack

>   *Still Lemonade with Lecithin

DAY 5

Breakfast

    4 *Devilled-Salmon Egg halves
    2 1-gram crisp breads (GG is an example)
    *Spiced Iced Decaf Coffee

Lunch

    *Fresh Tuna and Avocado Salad
    *Spicy Cocktail

Dinner

    *Japanese Egg Custard Soup
    *Oriental Prawns
    Tea or decaffeinated coffee with 15 ml cream and sugar substitute

Snack

    Cheese cubes

DAY 6

Breakfast

    *Spicy Sausage Omelette
    Tea or decaffeinated coffee with 15 ml cream and sugar substitute

Lunch

    *U.S. Hamburgers
    Tossed green salad with *Our Favorite Roquefort Dressing
    Diet soda or artificially sweetened iced tea

Dinner

    *Gourmet Poussins
    *Crispy White Radish
    Tea or decaffeinated coffee with 15 ml cream and sugar substitute

Snack

    *Vanilla Ice Cream

DAY 7

Breakfast

Steak and *Scrambled Eggs with 30 ml *Cheese Sauce
Tea or decaffeinated coffee with 15 ml cream and sugar substitute

Lunch

*Cold Avocado Soup
Tuna in olive oil with lemon wedge
½ cucumber, sliced
2 tablespoons *Mustard Vinaigrette
Tea or decaffeinated coffee with 15ml cream and sugar substitute

Dinner

*Prawns Parmesan
Tossed salad with *Tomato Dressing

Snack

*Mocha Drink

The Ongoing Weight-Loss Diet

DAY 1

Breakfast

> *Two-Cheese Omelette
> 3 rashers bacon (nitrate-free)
> 1 slice *4 Grain and Seed Bread
> Tea or decaffeinated coffee with 15 ml cream and sugar substitute

Lunch

> *Aubergine Parmigiana
> Tossed green salad with *Italian Dressing
> *Orange Cooler

Dinner

> *Caribbean Crab Balls
> *Halibut Roll-Ups
> *Broccoli in Cheese Sauce
> Tea or decaffeinated coffee with 15 ml cream and sugar substitute

Snack

> 2 squares of *Chocolate Fudge
> Diet soft drink

DAY 2

Breakfast

> *Poached Eggs on ham with 30 ml *Hollandaise Sauce
> 2 slices *4 Grain and Seed Bread
> Tea or decaffeinated coffee with 15 ml cream and sugar substitute

Lunch

> *Chicken Salad
> 6 fried pork rinds
> Diet soda or artificially sweetened iced tea

Dinner

*Enchiladas
Tossed green salad with *Dressing of the House
*Raspberry Rapture Ice Cream
Tea or decaffeinated coffee with 15 ml cream and sugar substitute

Snack

*Spiced Iced Decaf Coffee
2 *Peanut Butter Cookies

DAY 3

Breakfast

*Crab and Mushroom Omelette
2 slices *Rye Bread with cream cheese
Tea or decaffeinated coffee with 15 ml cream and sugar substitute

Lunch

*Dr. Atkins' Fromage Burger
½ tomato, sliced
¼ cucumber, sliced
Diet soda

Dinner

*New England Fish Chowder
*Tarragon Lobster Tails
*Porcini Mushrooms
*Raspberry Sorbet
Tea or decaffeinated coffee with 15 ml cream and sugar substitute

Snack

2 *Almond Ball Cookies

DAY 4

Breakfast

*Rye Bread, smoked salmon and cream cheese
2 slices onion
Tea or decaffeinated coffee with 15 ml cream and sugar substitute

Lunch

*Ham and Artichoke Omelette
Tossed green salad with *Basic French Dressing
1 slice *Cheese Cake
Iced decaffeinated coffee with cream

Dinner

*Fran's Special Pâté
Roast Beef with *Frozen Horseradish Cream
Chicory with *Parmesan Caesar Dressing
Tea or decaffeinated coffee with 15 ml cream and sugar substitute

Snack

125 ml *Decaf-Coffee Ice Cream

DAY 5

Breakfast

*Two-Cheese Omelette
4 slices crisp bacon
2 slices *4 Grain and Seed Bread

Lunch

*Vegetable Stock with *Dumplings
*Zucchini Stuffed with Cream Sauce
Romaine (Cos) Lettuce with *Mustard Vinaigrette
Diet soda

Dinner

*Sardine Snack stuffed into celery sticks
*Fennel Red Snapper
*Chic Asparagus

Tea or decaffeinated coffee with 15 ml cream and sugar substitute

Snack

2 *Brownie Squares

DAY 6

Breakfast

*Cappuccino
*Scrambled Eggs with ham and *Mustard Sauce
1 slice *Rye Bread with cream cheese
Tea or decaffeinated coffee with 15 ml cream and sugar substitute

Lunch

*Salad Niçoise with Fresh Tuna
*Orange Cooler

Dinner

*Tricolour Salad with Three Cheeses
*Chicken à la Firenze
½ small tomato, sliced
Tea or decaffeinated coffee with 15 ml cream and sugar substitute

Snack

Prepared sugar-free jelly with 15 ml of cream, whipped

DAY 7

Breakfast

Smoked whitefish or salmon with spring onion cream cheese on 2
slices *Rye Bread
*Scrambled Eggs
Tea or decaffeinated coffee with 15 ml cream and sugar substitute

Lunch

*U.S. Hamburgers with 1 slice of onion and lettuce
*Chocolate Shake

Dinner

>*Cream of Shiitake Mushroom Soup
>*Chicken Croquettes served on spaghetti squash
>Tossed green salad with *Dill Vinaigrette Dressing

Snack

>*Butter Pecan Ice Cream
>Diet soda

The Premaintenance Diet

DAY 1

Breakfast

> *Turkey Sausage
> Scrambled Eggs
> 2 slices *Courgette Bread

Lunch

> *Crunchy Seafood Salad
> *Vanilla Ice Cream
> Diet soda

Dinner

> ¼ cantaloupe with lemon slice
> *Stuffed Steak
> *Ratatouille
> *Lemon-Lime Mousse
> Tea or decaffeinated coffee with 15 ml cream and sugar substitute

Snack

> 20 macadamia nuts or
> 125 ml *Coconut Macadamia Ice Cream

DAY 2

Breakfast

*Aubergine and Cheddar Omelette
125 g broiled ham
2 slices *Rye Bread

Lunch

*Fresh Tuna and Avocado Salad
3 1-gram crisp breads (GG is an example)
*Fresh Lemonade with Lecithin

Dinner

*Manicotti
*Green Bean Chokes
*Tomato Lemon Aspic on lettuce leaves
Tea or decaffeinated coffee with 15 ml cream and sugar substitute

Snack

60 g almonds

DAY 3

Breakfast

French toast made with 4 slices *4 Grain and Seed Bread dipped
into a beaten egg and fried in butter
4 rashers of crisp bacon
Tea or decaffeinated coffee with 15 ml cream and sugar substitute

Lunch

*Hot Beef Salad
*Orange Cooler

Dinner

*Cannelloni
180 g steamed broccoli
Tossed salad with *Tomato Mayonnaise
*Italian Rum Cake
Tea or decaffeinated coffee with 15 ml cream and sugar substitute

Snack

> 30 g fresh raspberries and 30 ml whipped cream

DAY 4

Breakfast

> Your favorite cut of steak, sliced
> *Scrambled Eggs with *Hot Barbecue Sauce
> Tea or decaffeinated coffee with 15 ml cream and sugar substitute

Lunch

> *Salad Niçoise With Fresh Tuna
> 2 slices *Rye Bread and butter
> Diet soda
> *Confetti Mould

Dinner

> *Enchiladas
> Tossed green salad with *Creamy Celery Dressing
> *The Most Delicious Cucumbers
> Tea or decaffeinated coffee with 15 ml cream and sugar substitute

Snack

> 125 ml *Decaf-Coffee Ice Cream

DAY 5

Breakfast

> Smoked salmon, onion and eggs, scrambled
> 2 slices *Courgette Bread with spring onion cream cheese
> Tea or decaffeinated coffee with 15ml cream and sugar substitute

Lunch

> *Aubergine "Little Shoes"
> Tossed green salad with *Italian Dressing
> Tea or decaffeinated coffee with 15 ml cream and sugar substitute

Dinner

*Fish Stock with *Dumplings
*Sun Luck Scallops
*Chic Asparagus
Tea or decaffeinated coffee with 15 ml cream and sugar substitute

Snack

3 *Almond Ball Cookies

DAY 6

Breakfast

*Prawn and Goat Cheese Omelette
2 slices *4 Grain and Seed Bread
Tea or decaffeinated coffee with 15 ml cream and sugar substitute

Lunch

*Poached Salmon Salad
3 1-gram crisp breads (GG is an example)
Tea or decaffeinated coffee with 15 ml cream and sugar substitute

Dinner

*Cauliflower Soup with Dill and Caraway
*Gourmet Pork Chops
*String Beans Almandine
*Crispy White Radish
Tea or decaffeinated coffee with 15 ml cream and sugar substitute

Snack

125 ml *Maple Walnut Ice Cream

DAY 7

Breakfast

    *Peaches and Cream Omelette
    *Hot Chocolate

Lunch

    ¹/₂ cantaloupe stuffed with *Moulded Roquefort Spread
    *Tuna Loaf
    Iced tea or iced decaf coffee

Dinner

    *Roast Turkey With Almond Stuffing
    *Baked Spinach
    125 ml *Peach Melba Frozen Yoghurt
    Tea or decaffeinated coffee with 15 ml cream and sugar substitute

Snack

    60 g pecans (about 20)

The Yeast-Free Diet

The Yeast-Free Diet has food restrictions that the other diets do not have. Therefore, it is necessary to begin with a list of yeast no-no's. To learn more about how yeast affects your body, see page 15.

DO NOT EAT OR DRINK

Alcoholic beverages
Barbecue sauce
Bread or hamburger buns
Buttermilk
Cake
Cashews
Catsup
Cheeses (except fresh)
Chili peppers
Citric acid
Dried roasted nuts
Fruit (especially dried and
    cured)
Horseradish
Mayonnaise
Malted products
Milk

Mincemeat
Mushrooms
Pastry
Peanuts
Pickles
Pistachios
Pretzels
Rolls
Root beer
Sauerkraut
Smoked foods
Soured cream
Soy sauce
Sugars of any type
Tomato sauce or ketchup
Vitamins in a yeast base

This list may seem overwhelming. It is not! As you will see, this book is filled with wonderful recipes that will delight the taste buds and give a feeling of well-being.

Happily being faithful to this diet has very positive results. You will be able to overcome (with the help of supplements) your yeast sensitivity and once again enjoy—in moderation—foods containing yeast.

DAY 1

Breakfast

> 2–3 Eggs *Poached, *Hard or Soft Boiled
> 6 cooked prawns
> *Lemon Barbecue Sauce
> Tea or decaffeinated coffee with 15 ml cream and sugar substitute

Lunch

> *Gazpacho
> Tuna fish with *Vinegar-Free Mayonnaise
> 2 1-gram crisp breads (GG is an example)
> *Orange Cooler

Dinner

> *Spicy Spareribs
> Hearts of lettuce salad with *Tomato Mayonnaise Dressing
> Sugar-free jelly

Snack

> *Vanilla Ice Cream

DAY 2

Breakfast

> *Scrambled or *Sunny-Side Up and Over Easy eggs
> 3 slices boiled ham wrapped around a celery stick that is stuffed
> with cream cheese
> Tea or decaffeinated coffee with 15 ml cream and sugar substitute

Lunch

> *Brit Burger
> ½ cucumber, sliced, with minced fresh basil
> *Shape-Up Shake

Dinner

> *Lobster Tails with Tarragon
> *Crispy White Radish
> Tossed green salad with *Creamy Celery Seed Dressing made with

*Vinegar-Free Mayonnaise
Tea or decaffeinated coffee with 15 ml cream and sugar substitute

Snack

*Hot Mint Chocolate Nog

DAY 3

Breakfast

Sliced steak sautéed in garlic butter
$^{1}/_{2}$ small onion, raw or sautéed in butter
2 slices *4 Grain and Seed Bread
Tea or decaffeinated coffee with 15 ml cream and sugar substitute

Lunch

*Luncheon Omelette
*Mocha Drink

Dinner

*Sardine Snack on lettuce leaves
*Lemon-Basted Roast Chicken
Chicory with *Lime Dill Dressing

Snack

*Black and White Ice Cream Soda

DAY 4

Breakfast

*Herb Omelette
2 slices *4 Grain and Seed Bread with cream cheese
*Cappuccino

Lunch

*Chicken Salad Ham Roll made with fresh ham (always use
*Vinegar-Free Mayonnaise)
*Blender-Thick Raspberry Shake

Dinner

> *Japanese Egg Custard Soup (exclude mushrooms)
> *Oriental Prawns
> *Confetti Mould
> Tea or decaffeinated coffee with 15 ml cream and sugar substitute

Snack

> *Confetti Mould

DAY 5

Breakfast

> 4 *Devilled-Salmon Egg halves
> 2 slices *Rye Bread with butter
> *Spiced Iced Decaf Coffee

Lunch

> *U.S. Hamburgers with *Tomato Mayonnaise
> *Mock Potato Salad (exclude pickle)
> Diet soda

Dinner

> *Chicken Stock with *Dumplings
> *Gourmet Poussins
> Tossed green salad with *Basic Vinegar-Free Salad Dressing
> Tea or decaffeinated coffee with 15 ml cream and sugar substitute

Snack

> *Ice Lollies

DAY 6

Breakfast

>*Ham and Artichoke Omelette
2 slices *Rye Bread
Tea or decaffeinated coffee with 15 ml cream and sugar substitute

Lunch

>*Chicken Croquettes
Tossed green salad with *Tomato Mayonnaise
*Confetti Mould
Diet soda

Dinner

>*Klara's Aubergine Appetizer on celery rounds
*Curried Crab
Steamed broccoli
*Vanilla Ice Cream
Tea or decaffeinated coffee with 15 ml cream and sugar substitute

Snack

>Two *Brownie squares
Diet soda

DAY 7

Breakfast

>*Salmon Soufflé
2 slices *4 Grain and Seed Bread
Tea or decaffeinated coffee with 15 ml cream and sugar substitute

Lunch

>*Curry Burgers
Tossed green salad with *Lime Dill Dressing
2 *Almond Ball Cookies
Diet soda

Dinner

> *Chicken Cacciatore with spaghetti squash
> *String Beans Amandine
> *Lemon-Lime Mousse
> Tea or decaffeinated coffee with 15 ml cream and sugar substitute

Snack

> 125 ml *Decaf-Coffee Ice Cream

The Maintenance Diet

When you have reached your ideal weight, you will begin Maintenance. At this level you may choose freely from any recipe in the book. And you may add back pulses; all vegetables, including carrots, peas, beets, potatoes, sweet potatoes; all the sweet winter squash varieties and plaintains. Grains are permitted on the Maintenance Level. Actually you will be eating a very healthy diet. That is the good news.

Sugars of all types are excluded from all of our diets. Although some of you may think they taste good, sugars are destructive to your health. Therefore, sugars—including honey, molasses, maple sugar and syrup, fructose, beet sugar, barley malt sugar, glucose, maltose, dextrose, corn syrup, sorbitol, mannitol, and hexitol—still are and will always be the bad news.

We encourage you to eat more protein than carbohydrates, unless the condition of your health does not permit it. Please drink 6 to 8 glasses of water a day and see a nutritionist who can help you with a vitamin program specific to your needs. When this becomes your lifestyle, you will be the slim, healthy, and energetic person that you always aspired to be.

The Yeast-Free Maintenance Diet

This diet is much the same as the Maintenance Diet. However, on this diet you will restrict cheeses, vinegars, and all fermented foods as well as sugar. In addition, you may wish to ask for yeast-free products at your health food store.

4 | *Recipes*

Eggs

Eggs are the perfect protein and we recommend them, especially **free range, organic eggs**, available in health food stores. In most areas, these high-quality eggs are in supermarkets. The chickens that lay these eggs have not been injected with antibiotics or hormones and have not been fed chemicals. Always check the date on the box to ensure that the eggs are fresh.

You know that I don't have to tell you how to cook eggs. You have been cooking them for years. But I'd like to share some hints that have helped me. With any luck they may make your egg dishes even better than your usual great!

Separating An Egg:

Egg white will not whisk stiffly if one drop of yolk gets mixed with the white when you separate the eggs. You can remove a small drop of yolk from white by using the cracked egg shell. Just dip it into the white and remove the yolk.

Whisking Egg Whites:

To get the most volume from egg whites, bring them to room temperature before beating. They may be whisked with a wire whisk in a large metal bowl, a rotary beater, or an electric mixer. The electric mixer is most practical. Since egg whites lose volume quickly, whisk them just before you need them.

Adding a pinch of cream of tartar to the unwhisked whites will help them sustain stiffness.

When adding whisked egg whites to a recipe, fold them in with a rubber spatula being careful not to break them down.

Using Egg Yolks as Thickeners:

This book uses egg yolks to thicken sauces, ice creams and soufflés. Two egg yolks are equal to about 8.5 g (1 tablespoon) of flour or thickener. Beat eggs in a separate bowl and add 60 ml of sauce to be thickened to the bowl. Beat together well. When eggs are blended with sauce, add egg mixture to sauce—stirring constantly over a low flame until sauce thickens. Do not boil sauce or egg yolk will scramble and sauce will become lumpy.

Soft-Boiled Eggs

1 serving

2 large eggs, at room temperature
cold water to cover

Purchase a device called an "egg pricker" and put a small hole in the large end of the egg. This keeps eggs from cracking during cooking. Place eggs in water and bring to a boil. Boil for 3 minutes for loose eggs, 4 minutes for runny yolks and firmed whites, and 5 minutes for firmed yolks and whites. Run under cold water to stop cooking. Crack open tops and serve in egg cups.

GRAMS PER SERVING 1.2

Hard-Boiled Eggs

1 serving

2 large eggs, at room temperature
cold water to cover
Prick broad side of the egg. Place eggs in water. Bring water to a boil. Cover egg pan and turn off heat. Allow eggs to remain in water for 20 minutes. Refrigerate to cool.

GRAMS PER SERVING 1.2

How to Tell if an Egg Is Hard Boiled:
    Hard-boiled eggs will spin in their shells. Eggs that have not been cooked will not spin.

Scrambled Eggs

1 serving

2 eggs
1 tablespoon whipping cream
15 g unsalted butter
salt and pepper to taste

Break eggs into a small bowl. Add cream and beat well with a wire whisk. Melt butter in a non-stick frying pan, then add eggs. Cook on a low heat until eggs set. Season with salt and pepper (you may add other seasonings). When eggs set, "scramble" them with a fork. Slide out of pan and enjoy.
Variation: Sprinkle grated cheese over set eggs before scrambling.

GRAMS PER SERVING 1.6

Sunny-Side Up and Over Easy

1 serving

2 eggs
15 g unsalted butter
salt and pepper to taste

Melt butter in non-stick frying pan. Break eggs, one at a time, into a flat saucer and slide them into the pan. Cook on a low heat until whites become solidly white and centre is runny. If Sunny-Side Up is your preference, remove from pan to plate after about 2½ minutes. For Over Easy use a spatula or fish slice and carefully flip eggs over. Cook for 30 seconds more. Salt and pepper to taste.

GRAMS PER SERVING 1.2

Poached Eggs

1 serving

2 eggs, at room temperature
salt and pepper to taste

Fill a frying pan or saucepan halfway with water and heat to a simmer. Break eggs one at a time into a flat saucer. Slide into the simmering water, one at a time. Allow to simmer for 3 minutes until whites are no longer transparent. Remove from water with a slotted spoon. Place on a plate, season with salt and pepper and enjoy.

GRAMS PER SERVING 1.2

Cheese-Baked Eggs

1 serving

2 eggs, at room temperature
2 tablespoons grated Parmesan cheese
10 g unsalted butter
2 tablespoons whipping cream
salt and pepper to taste

Preheat oven to 190° C (gas 5).

Fill a baking dish halfway with boiling water. Divide the butter between 2 small ramekins. Carefully break an egg into each cup. Place 1 tablespoon of cream over each egg. Top with cheese, divided evenly. Place ramekins in water bath in baking pan and set in the oven. Bake for 10 minutes. Salt and pepper to taste.

GRAMS PER SERVING 2.4

Basic Omelette

2 servings

30 g butter
4 eggs
1 tablespoon whipping cream
½ teaspoon seasoned salt
freshly cracked pepper to taste

Melt butter in a non-stick frying pan or omelette pan. Tilt pan to cover well with butter.

Beat eggs with cream, salt and pepper. Pour into pan and tilt pan to spread eggs to edges of pan.

Cook over a low flame until eggs begin to set. Loosen eggs from sides of pan with a spatula. Tilt pan again to allow uncooked eggs to run to the sides. Carefully fold outer edges of omelette into the centre to resemble a flat cone. Slide omelette out of pan and serve.

When filling omelette, spoon mixture on to centre of omelette before folding edges into the centre.

TOTAL GRAMS 2.8
GRAMS PER SERVING 1.4

Bacon and Onion Omelette

2 servings

9 rashers streaky bacon
40 g chopped onion
1 Basic Omelette recipe

Cut bacon into small pieces. Fry in small frying pan until crisp. Add onion and sauté until translucent. Pour off fat. Follow method for making *Basic Omelette,* above.

Place bacon and onion in centre of omelette before folding over. Fold over and cook 1 minute. Serve immediately.

TOTAL GRAMS 6.0
GRAMS PER SERVING 3.0

Cheese-Tease Omelette

4 servings

8 eggs
100 g cottage cheese
120 g full fat soft (cream) cheese, softened
pinch salt
2–4 teaspoons sugar substitute, to taste
1 teaspoon vanilla essence
½ teaspoon ground cinnamon
60 ml whipping cream
45 g butter
2 tablespoons soured cream (optional)

Combine all ingredients except butter and soured cream in a bowl and beat with a wire whisk or mixer until smooth.

Melt butter in a large non-stick omelette pan. Follow method for making *Basic Omelette.*

Slide out of pan and serve plain or garnished with soured cream.

TOTAL GRAMS 19.8
GRAMS PER SERVING 5.0

Peaches and Cream Omelette

4 servings

225 g full fat soft (cream) cheese, softened
8 eggs
pinch salt
60 ml whipping cream
1–2 teaspoons sugar substitute
30 g butter
5 tablespoons chopped Poached Peaches *(p. 215)*

Combine all ingredients except butter and chopped peaches in a bowl and beat until smooth.

Cook according to instructions for *Basic Omelette* (p. 48).

When centre is firm, spoon peaches on to the centre, fold over sides.

Slide out of pan and serve.

TOTAL GRAMS 18.7
GRAMS PER SERVING 4.7

Aubergine and Cheddar Omelette

4 servings

80 g peeled and cubed aubergine
4 tablespoons virgin olive oil
1 clove garlic, chopped (or ¼ teaspoon garlic powder)
125 ml prepared tomato sauce or passata
8 eggs, beaten
½ teaspoon seasoned salt
60 g Cheddar cheese, grated

Soak the aubergine cubes in a bowl of cold water for ½ hour. Drain and dry well.

Place 3 tablespoons of the olive oil in a frying pan. Add aubergine and garlic or garlic powder. Sauté until aubergine begins to brown. Add tomato sauce or passata and heat through. Set aside.

Heat remaining 1 tablespoon oil in large frying pan. Add eggs, salt and cheese. Continue to cook over low heat until they set.

Spoon aubergine mixture on to centre of omelette, fold over sides.

TOTAL GRAMS 19.4
GRAMS PER SERVING 4.8

Herb Omelette

2 servings

4 eggs
1 tablespoon chopped chives
1 tablespoon finely chopped dill
2 tablespoons mascarpone cheese
30 g butter
seasoned salt to taste

Combine all ingredients; beat until smooth and thoroughly combined.
Cook according to instructions for *Basic Omelette*.

TOTAL GRAMS 4.1
GRAMS PER SERVING 2.0

Eggs Florentine

6 servings

225 g fresh spinach (or 280 g frozen spinach)
6 eggs
seasoned salt
1 recipe Cheese Sauce *(p. 186)*

Preheat oven to 180° C/gas 4.
Cook spinach in a medium saucepan over low heat. Drain well.
Chop fine.
Place hot spinach in shallow baking dish.
Make a depression for each egg in spinach. Break one egg into
each depression. Salt to taste.
Prepare cheese sauce. Pour over eggs and spinach. Bake for 25
minutes.

TOTAL GRAMS 29.7
GRAMS PER SERVING 5.0

Salmon Soufflé

6 servings

30 g butter
3 tablespoons soy flour
1 teaspoon seasoned salt
250 ml whipping cream, heated
250 g salmon fillet, poached, or canned, boned and drained
seasoned salt and cayenne pepper to taste
3 eggs, separated
4 teaspoons lemon juice

Preheat oven to 200° C/gas 6.

Prepare soufflé dish by greasing bottom and sides with half the butter. Place in refrigerator until ready to use.

Melt remaining butter over low heat and stir in flour and salt. Whisk vigorously for 1 full minute to avoid floury taste. Add heated cream and continue cooking, whisking constantly until thickened. Remove from heat and cool.

Add salmon, salt and cayenne. Beat egg yolks and blend them into the sauce mixture.

Stiffly whisk egg whites and fold into salmon mixture with lemon juice. Pour mixture into soufflé dish.

Set in a pan filled with 7.5 cm of hot water and bake about 35 minutes until firm and puffed. Serve immediately.

TOTAL GRAMS 14.9
GRAMS PER SERVING 2.5

Spicy Sausage Bake

4 servings

225 g spicy sausage, cut in bite-size pieces
1 clove garlic, finely chopped
60 ml olive oil
1 teaspoon seasoned salt
1 teaspoon caraway seeds
1 tablespoon tomato purée
2 drops Tabasco sauce, or to taste
6 eggs, beaten
1 tablespoon grated Parmesan cheese

Preheat oven to 170° C gas 3.

Sauté sausage and garlic in olive oil until sausage is well browned. Drain off fat. Add salt, caraway seeds, tomato purée and Tabasco sauce. Stir well. Cool. Combine eggs and Parmesan cheese. Spoon meat mixture into baking dish and cover with eggs. Bake for 45 minutes or until set.

TOTAL GRAMS 11.4
GRAMS PER SERVING 2.9

Luncheon Omelette

4 servings

2 tablespoons olive oil
6 shiitake mushrooms, thinly sliced
4 spring onions, thinly sliced
12 sugar snap peas, trimmed
2 slices sun-dried tomatoes, diced
6 eggs
2 tablespoons whipping cream
1 tablespoon finely chopped dill (or 1 teaspoon dried)
30 g unsalted butter
30 g herby goat cheese
salt and pepper to taste

Heat olive oil in a frying pan over medium heat. Sauté mushrooms and spring onions for 2 minutes. Add sugar snap peas and sun-dried tomatoes. Cook for 3 minutes (peas will remain crunchy).

Whisk eggs with cream and dill; pour carefully over vegetables. Dot centre of omelette with goat cheese and butter. Fold over sides. Season with salt and pepper.

TOTAL GRAMS 34.6
GRAMS PER SERVING 8.7

Two-Cheese Omelette

2 servings

30 g unsalted butter
2 tablespoons finely chopped onion
4 eggs
2 tablespoons whipping cream
120 g soft cheese, mashed or chopped
60 g firm cheese, grated
1 tablespoon chopped parsley

This omelette is delicious when you choose one hard and one soft cheese such as cream cheese and Cheddar or Camembert and Parmesan. Use the soft cheese to mix with the egg mixture and the hard cheese in the centre of the omelette.

Heat butter in a non-stick frying pan over medium heat. Add onion and cook until transparent. Beat eggs with cream and soft-textured cheese. Pour into pan. Spread egg mixture by tilting pan. Cook until eggs set. Sprinkle grated hard cheese over eggs. Cook 1 minute. Slice egg pancake in two. Fold each semicircle in half. Flip over to melt cheese and brown both sides. Serve hot and crisp. Garnish with parsley.

TOTAL GRAMS 7.2
GRAMS PER SERVING 3.6

Crab and Mushroom Omelette

6 servings

30 g butter
6 shiitake mushrooms, thinly sliced
2 tablespoons chopped spring onion
110 g white crab meat
1 tablespoon sherry
6 eggs
45 ml whipping cream

Melt butter in non-stick frying pan. Add mushrooms and onion and sauté until light brown. Stir in crab meat.

Simmer for 3 minutes. Add sherry and simmer 1 minute more. Remove half of crab mixture.

Beat eggs and cream together. Pour carefully over crab mixture in pan. Cook until set.

Place remaining crab mixture over top of omelette after it has been folded.

TOTAL GRAMS 21.8
GRAMS PER SERVING 3.6

Ham and Artichoke Omelette

4 servings

1 × 180-g jar marinated artichoke hearts, drained
2 tablespoons grated Parmesan cheese
8 eggs
3 tablespoons mascarpone cheese
seasoned salt and pepper to taste
120 g ham, thinly sliced

Use a large non-stick omelette pan.

Place artichoke hearts on kitchen paper and pat oil off. Roll hearts in Parmesan cheese; set aside. Beat eggs, mascarpone cheese, and salt and pepper together in a bowl until smooth. Follow the *Basic Omelette* instructions for cooking on page 48. When egg mixture is set, cover surface with ham slices. Place artichoke hearts in centre and fold sides over. Slice in four pieces before removing from pan, and serve.

TOTAL GRAMS 18.7
GRAMS PER SERVING 9.4

Prawn and Goat Cheese Omelette

2 servings

8 raw prawns, shelled and de-veined
4 tablespoons garlic oil
30 g unsalted butter
4 eggs
60 g herbed goat cheese, crumbled
4 sun-dried tomato halves softened in olive oil, finely chopped

Use a 23 cm non-stick frying pan or omelette pan.

Butterfly prawns by cutting ³/₄ of the way through—along the back vein. Open prawn to resemble a butterfly.

Sear the prawns in hot garlic oil (about 2 minutes on each side). Remove to kitchen paper. Wipe oil from pan.

Add butter to pan. Beat eggs with goat cheese and follow the *Basic Omelette* instructions for cooking on page 48.

When eggs are set, place prawns and sun-dried tomatoes on egg pancake and fold over.

TOTAL GRAMS 15.4
GRAMS PER SERVING 7.7

Appetizers

Marbled Tea Eggs From China

12 egg halves

6 eggs
30 ml soy sauce
2 tablespoons salt
3 tablespoons black tea
1 tablespoon anise essence

Cover eggs with cold water and bring to a boil. Reduce heat and simmer 10 minutes.

Remove eggs, cool, and crack the shells in several places, but do not peel.

Bring 1 litre of water to a boil. Add remaining ingredients and eggs. Simmer for one hour. Cool.

Place eggs, still in the liquid, in the refrigerator. Leave overnight.

To serve, shell eggs and cut in half. They are very attractive on the hors d'oeuvres tray.

TOTAL GRAMS 5.2
GRAMS PER SERVING 0.4

Deviled-Salmon Eggs

12 egg halves

6 eggs
3 tablespoons mayonnaise
125 g boneless cooked, flaked salmon, canned or smoked
½ teaspoon lemon juice
1 teaspoon Dijon mustard
1 teaspoon Worcestershire sauce
½ teaspoon salt
dash of pepper

Cover eggs with cold water and bring to a boil. Reduce heat and simmer gently for 15 minutes, turning often to help keep yolks in centre. Run eggs under cold water and remove shells. Slice eggs in half lengthways. Remove yolks.

Mash yolks and mayonnaise together until smooth. Add remaining ingredients and mix well.

Spoon mixture into egg whites.

Garnish with additional pieces of salmon if desired. Refrigerate for at least ½ hour before serving.

TOTAL GRAMS 5.7
GRAMS PER SERVING 0.5

Swedish Meatballs

8 meatballs

60 ml whipping cream
60 ml water
20 g sugar-free fried pork rinds, crushed
110 g minced beef
110 g minced pork
110 g minced veal
1 large onion, finely chopped
40 g butter
2 teaspoons seasoned salt
1 recipe Cream Sauce *(page 180)*
½ teaspoon grated nutmeg
1 teaspoon caraway seeds

Mix cream and water together in a small bowl. Add crushed pork rinds and allow to soak until softened, about 10 minutes. Combine beef, pork and veal.

Mix cream mixture, meats and onion together. Add seasoned salt. Shape into small balls, and brown in butter in a medium frying pan over medium heat.

Remove balls to chafing dish and keep warm.

Make *Cream Sauce* and pour over meatballs. Garnish with nutmeg and caraway seeds.

TOTAL GRAMS 7.0
GRAMS PER SERVING 0.9

Turkey Meatballs

8 meatballs

30 g butter
1 small onion, finely chopped
1 medium celery stick, finely chopped
1 clove garlic, finely chopped
225 g minced turkey
1 teaspoon seasoned salt
¼ teaspoon grated Parmesan cheese
½ teaspoon dried thyme
1 egg
¼ teaspoon curry powder

Heat butter in a medium frying pan. Sauté onion, celery and garlic until golden brown.

Place turkey in a bowl, add onion mixture and remaining ingredients. Mix well with a fork. Shape into 2.5-cm balls and sauté until well-browned.

TOTAL GRAMS 10.4
GRAMS PER SERVING 1.3

Salami and Parmesan

8 cubes

225 g salami, cut into eight cubes
2 eggs, beaten
50 g grated Parmesan cheese
walnut or peanut oil, for frying

Dip salami cubes into beaten eggs. Roll in Parmesan cheese until coated.
   Repeat.
   Deep fry in hot oil for 30 seconds, until lightly browned.

TOTAL GRAMS 7.0
GRAMS PER SERVING 0.9

Heavenly Wings

Hors d'oeuvres for 6

750 g chicken wings, about twelve
250 ml Tamari soy sauce
2 tablespoons sugar substitute
60 ml white wine
2 cloves garlic, mashed
60 ml sesame oil
½ teaspoon ground ginger

Rinse wings and pat dry. Cut into pieces at joints. Discard wing tips. Combine remaining ingredients.
   Spread wings in shallow baking dish. Do not overlap. Pour sauce over wings. Marinate overnight in refrigerator. Preheat oven to 170° C (gas 3). Bake in marinade for 1½ hours.

TOTAL GRAMS 19.9
GRAMS PER SERVING 3.3

Sardine Snack

3 snacks

1 × 90-g can skinless and boneless sardines, drained
½ teaspoon dried parsley
¼ teaspoon dried dill
3 hard-boiled eggs, mashed
¼ teaspoon salt
180 g soft (cream) cheese, softened
20 g chopped onion
¾ teaspoon lemon juice

Combine all ingredients in a blender or food processor. Blend until smooth. Serve, well chilled, on bed of lettuce leaves.

TOTAL GRAMS 7.1
GRAMS PER SERVING 2.4

Soured Cream Clam Dip

8 servings

250 ml soured cream
1 × 200-g can chopped clams, drained, reserving 1 tablespoon juice
1 tablespoon grated onion
1 teaspoon celery seed
4 tablespoons mayonnaise
1 tablespoon lemon juice
seasoned salt and pepper to taste
1 tablespoon Worcestershire sauce

Mix all ingredients together well. Refrigerate for at least 1 hour. Serve with vegetables or fried pork rinds.

TOTAL GRAMS 30.2
GRAMS PER SERVING 3.8

Guacamole

8 60-ml servings

1 avocado, peeled and chopped
80 g onion, chopped
1 tomato, chopped
⅓ cucumber, peeled and chopped
½ teaspoon paprika
½ teaspoon seasoned salt
1 jalapeño pepper, finely chopped
⅛ teaspoon hot chilli flakes
1 tablespoon soured cream
1 tablespoon chopped parsley

Place avocado, onion, tomato and cucumber in the work bowl of a food processor and process 10 seconds. Season with paprika, salt, and peppers. Add soured cream and parsley. Process 5 seconds. Refrigerate. Use as dip with sliced cucumbers.

TOTAL GRAMS 34.6
GRAMS PER SERVING 4.3

Fran's Special Pâté

20 slices

4 rashers nitrate-free bacon
450 g chicken livers
600–700 g skinless chicken breast fillet, pounded flat
4 teaspoons seasoned salt
3 tablespoons bacon fat
2 tablespoons butter
2 tablespoons white wine
½ 230-g can water chestnuts, drained
2 hard-boiled eggs
1 Boursin cheese, about 90 g
3 tablespoons sweet basil
freshly ground black pepper

Preheat oven to 140° C (gas 1).

Cook bacon until crisp. Reserve fat.

Place 2 tablespoons of bacon fat in frying pan. Sauté chicken livers about 5 minutes over medium heat. Remove from pan and set aside.

Add butter to pan and melt over medium heat; add chicken breast and sauté in butter for 3 minutes on each side. Add wine and simmer for 3 minutes.

Place cooked bacon, chicken livers, chicken breast, water chestnuts and eggs into a large wooden chopping bowl or food processor and chop fine.

Add seasoned salt, reserved bacon fat, Boursin cheese, basil and pepper. Mix well. Pack into a large buttered deep rectangular dish or loaf tin. Place a heavy weight on top to keep pâté from rising.

Bake for 2 hours. Turn oven off and allow pâté to remain undisturbed until oven is cold. Remove from oven and refrigerate. Unmould and cut into slices.

TOTAL GRAMS 29.6
GRAMS PER 1-SLICE SERVING 1.5

Cheesy Ham Snack

6 servings

1 tablespoon mayonnaise
1 tablespoon grated Parmesan cheese
6 slices Black Forest ham
1 small tomato, sliced thin
6 thin slices Swiss cheese

Mix mayonnaise with Parmesan cheese.

Spread mixture on slices of ham, top with tomato slices. Roll up. Place ham rolls on thin slices of Swiss cheese and roll again. Fasten with cocktail sticks.

TOTAL GRAMS 9.4
GRAMS PER SERVING 1.6

Caribbean Crab Balls

30 canapés

30 g butter
2 tablespoons (20 g) chopped onion
1 clove garlic, finely chopped
40 g grated coconut, or unsweetened desiccated coconut
450 g white crab meat, fresh or canned
1 egg, beaten
30 ml whipping cream
2 teaspoons curry powder
1 teaspoon salt
40 g sugar-free fried pork rinds, crushed
125 ml oil

Melt the butter in medium frying pan over medium heat. Sauté onion and garlic until transparent.

Add coconut to pan and sauté until light brown. Remove from heat and cool.

In a separate bowl, combine crab meat, egg, cream, curry powder and salt. Add onion, garlic and coconut mixture. Mix well.

Shape into 2.5-cm balls. Roll in pork rinds. Heat oil in frying pan. Brown crabmeat balls in hot oil. Drain thoroughly on kitchen paper. Serve on cocktail sticks.

TOTAL GRAMS 20.3
GRAMS PER SERVING   0.7

Klara's Aubergine Appetizer

6 servings

1 medium aubergine
1 medium onion, sliced
1 tablespoon extra-virgin olive oil
1 teaspoon balsamic vinegar
¼ teaspoon seasoned salt
pepper to taste

Preheat oven to 180° C (gas 4). Bake aubergine for 1 hour until soft. Cool and peel. Mash aubergine until smooth and combine with remaining ingredients.

TOTAL GRAMS 38.3
GRAMS PER SERVING   7.0

Toasted Nuts

140 g toasted nuts

5 g butter
140 g nuts of your choice

Melt butter in non-stick pan. Stir in nuts and sauté until lightly browned. Place on kitchen paper to absorb excess oil.

If you like them salty, use seasoned salt to taste.
If you like them sweet, use a sugar substitute to taste.
If you like them spicy, use chilli powder to taste.

TOTAL GRAMS FOR TOASTED ALMONDS   5.8
TOTAL GRAMS FOR TOASTED WALNUTS   10.4
TOTAL GRAMS FOR TOASTED PECANS   5.2
TOTAL GRAMS FOR TOASTED PINE NUTS   8.0

Soups

These four stocks are important to many of the recipes in this book. They freeze easily and safely. I freeze them in small containers (no more than 500 ml) so they can be defrosted quickly. Once you've tried these stocks, their value will be apparent. Every recipe will taste much more zesty and flavourful as a result of using them.

Chicken Stock

10 250-ml servings

1 chicken, about 2 kg, rinsed
3 litres cold water
1 teaspoon seasoned salt
2 celery sticks, chopped
1 tablespoon chopped parsley
1 small onion, chopped
1 parsnip, diced
1 bay leaf
½ teaspoon dried thyme
1 chicken stock cube (preferably Knorr)

Place chicken in cold water in a large saucepan. Bring to a boil over medium heat. Skim off foam that forms on top of water, as the chicken cooks.

Add remaining ingredients, cover and simmer chicken until it is tender, about 1½ hours.

Cool. Remove chicken and strain stock. Chill the stock in a covered container in refrigerator.

Remove layer of fat that will rise to the top when thoroughly chilled.

Heat stock for soup and sauces. Or use it cold to make an aspic or jellied soup.

The chicken and vegetables may be returned to stock for a chicken soup meal or use chicken to make *Chicken Salad*, pages 85–86.

TOTAL GRAMS 19.8
GRAMS PER SERVING 2.0

Cream of Chicken Soup

1 serving

250 ml Chicken Stock *(page 69)*
30 ml whipping cream
1 egg yolk (for thickening)

Whisk cream and yolk until blended and whisk into hot stock. Simmer 1 minute. Do not boil!

TOTAL GRAMS 3.3

Vegetable Stock

8 250-ml servings

30 g butter
2 sprigs fresh parsley, or 1 teaspoon dried parsley
1 large onion, sliced
1 large carrot, sliced
3 celery sticks, sliced
2 litres water
6 whole peppercorns
2 whole cloves
1 bay leaf
2 tablespoons wine vinegar (optional)

Melt butter in deep saucepan over medium flame. Add vegetables and sauté for 5 minutes. Add water and seasonings, cover tightly, and simmer for 30 minutes.

Strain and use as directed in recipes.

TOTAL GRAMS 20.1
GRAMS PER SERVING 2.5

Beef Stock

10 250-ml servings

900 g stewing steak
1 teaspoon salt
3 litres cold water
¼ teaspoon ground pepper
80 g diced onion
60 g diced carrot
60 g diced celery
100 g diced tomato
1 teaspoon chopped parsley
10 g chopped green pepper

Place meat and salt in cold water, and bring to a boil over low heat. Skim foam off the top. Cover and simmer for 2½ hours.

Add the vegetables, seasonings and pepper and cook slowly for an additional 1½ hours.

Remove meat and serve with horseradish or mustard sauce. Strain stock and use as directed in recipes.

TOTAL GRAMS 15.3
GRAMS PER SERVING 1.5

Fish Stock

8 250-ml servings

900 g fish and/or fish bones (not oily fish)
2 litres water
2 cloves
½ teaspoon mace blades
3 celery sticks, with tops, diced
1 sprig parsley, chopped
1 bay leaf
5 peppercorns
1 tablespoon salt

Place all ingredients in deep saucepan. Cover tightly and bring to a boil. Lower flame and simmer gently for 45 minutes. Strain, cool, and store in refrigerator. Use as directed in recipes.

TOTAL GRAMS 5.4
GRAMS PER SERVING 0.7

Dumpling Soup

4 servings

15 g soft butter
1 egg plus 1 yolk
125 ml whipping cream
pinch of grated nutmeg
1 litre Chicken Stock *(page 69)*

Grease bottom and sides of the top of a double boiler with butter.

Beat egg, egg yolk, cream, salt and nutmeg together with fork. Pour into top of double boiler.

Cook over hot (not boiling) water for 45 minutes, or until set and firm. Turn out on to greaseproof or parchment paper and cool. Slice into cubes. Add to clear hot stock. Serve immediately.

TOTAL GRAMS 13.3
GRAMS PER SERVING 3.3

Cream of Shiitake Mushroom Soup

10 servings

225 g shiitake mushrooms, sliced thin
½ medium onion, finely chopped
120 g butter
1 litre Chicken Stock *(page 69)*
1 litre Beef Stock *(page 71)*
2 tablespoons toasted sesame seeds
½ teaspoon seasoned salt

250 ml whipping cream
1 tablespoon minced chives

Sauté mushrooms and onions in half the butter for 5 minutes over medium heat. Mix the stocks; add mushrooms and onions.

Add crushed sesame seeds and remaining butter; heat stirring until butter melts.

Add salt. Cook over low heat for 10 minutes. Cool slightly. Stir in cream until well blended. Do not allow to boil.

Serve warm or cold, garnished with chives.

TOTAL GRAMS 44.6
GRAMS PER SERVING   4.5

Creamy Ricotta Soup

6 servings

1 onion, chopped fine
1 celery stick, chopped
2 green peppers, chopped
40 g butter
750 ml Vegetable Stock (page 70)
1½ teaspoon seasoned salt
½ teaspoon paprika
500 g ricotta cheese, sieved
4 sprigs parsley, minced
3 rashers streaky bacon, fried crisp and crumbled

Sauté onion, celery and peppers in butter in a deep saucepan. Add vegetable stock, seasoned salt and paprika.

Cover and simmer gently for 1 hour over low heat.

Add ricotta cheese and blend well. If greater smoothness is desired, put mixture in blender; blend at medium speed until smooth.

Garnish with parsley and crumbled bacon. Serve hot.

TOTAL GRAMS 40.2
GRAMS PER SERVING   6.7

Gazpacho

6 servings

¼ *teaspoon garlic powder*
1 onion, chopped
4 sprigs parsley, chopped
30 ml wine vinegar
45 ml olive oil
¼ *teaspoon cayenne pepper*
¼ *teaspoon seasoned salt*
375 ml Chicken Stock *(page 69)*
4 large tomatoes, peeled and chopped
½ *cucumber, peeled, de-seeded, and diced*
2 tablespoons crushed sugar-free fried pork rinds (optional)

Place all ingredients in blender or food processor. Blend until smooth. Chill overnight. Serve in chilled bowls. Garnish each with additional cucumber, pepper and crushed pork rinds, as desired.

TOTAL GRAMS 43.2
GRAMS PER SERVING 7.2

Cold Avocado Soup

6 servings

1 avocado (about 500 g), peeled and diced
45 ml lime juice
½ teaspoon salt
dash pepper
dash nutmeg
750 ml Chicken Stock *(page 69)*
60 ml whipping cream, whipped

Place avocado, lime juice, salt, pepper and nutmeg in a blender. Add 125 ml *Chicken Stock*. Blend 30 seconds at high speed. Pour into bowl.

Whisk in remaining stock and chill until icy cold.

Serve garnished with a spoonful of whipped cream and a sprinkle of nutmeg.

TOTAL GRAMS 31.3
GRAMS PER SERVING 5.2

Japanese Egg Custard Soup

6 servings

140 g julienne-cut cooked chicken or diced raw, peeled prawns
3 water chestnuts, diced
6 mushrooms, diced
2 spring onions, chopped
1 tablespoon sherry
4 eggs, beaten
1 teaspoon salt
750 ml Beef Stock *(page 71)*
12 spinach or lettuce leaves

Preheat oven to 150° C (gas 2).

Combine chicken or prawns, water chestnuts, mushrooms, spring onions and sherry.

Divide mixture evenly among 6 ramekins or custard cups.

Beat eggs, salt and stock together. Pour into ramekins or custard cups. Cover with spinach or lettuce leaves.

Place in large pan with about 7 cm boiling water. Cover pan and bake for 30 minutes or until mixture is set.

TOTAL GRAMS 16.5
GRAMS PER SERVING 2.8

New England Fish Chowder

6 servings

900 g cod fillets
4 rashers bacon, diced
1 small onion, chopped
2 tablespoons chopped parsley
500 ml Fish Stock (page 71)
1 bay leaf
1 teaspoon seasoned salt
pepper to taste
500 ml whipping cream

Cut fish fillets into 2.5-cm cubes. Place bacon in deep saucepan over low heat and sauté until golden brown. Add onions and sauté until transparent. Add parsley and cook 1 minute more.

Add stock, bay leaf, salt and pepper. Cover and cook for a few minutes to combine flavours. Add fish, and simmer for 10 minutes. Add cream and heat just until heated through. Do not boil. Serve immediately.

TOTAL GRAMS 20.4
GRAMS PER SERVING 3.4

New England Clam Chowder

6 servings

Wash 3 dozen clams thoroughly. Steam in covered pot in 10-15 cm boiling water until shells open (no longer than 5 minutes). Strain clam stock and use as part of liquid in recipe. Chop clams coarsely and substitute for cod fillets in *New England Fish Chowder,* page 76.

TOTAL GRAMS 33.6
GRAMS PER SERVING 5.6

Baked Scallop and Fish Soup

4 servings

30 g unsalted butter
1 large fish fillet, any variety
2 cloves garlic, minced
3 small ripe tomatoes, peeled and chopped
½ medium onion, chopped
10 shiitake mushrooms, or any mushrooms, sliced thin
70 g pine kernels
450 g scallops
60 ml white wine
1 tablespoon chopped dill, or 1 teaspoon dried dill

Preheat oven to 180° C (gas 4).
     Melt butter on bottom of a deep-sided baking dish.
     Place fish in dish and top with garlic. Add tomato, onion, mushrooms, nuts and scallops. Sprinkle with wine. Cover and bake for 20 minutes. Remove cover and cook 10 minutes more. Place in soup bowls. Garnish with dill.

TOTAL GRAMS 58.0
GRAMS PER SERVING 14.5

Cauliflower Soup with Dill and Caraway

6 servings

30 g unsalted butter
3 leeks (white part only), chopped
½ medium cauliflower, chopped
750 ml Chicken Stock *(page 69)*
1 chicken stock cube
250 ml whipping cream
2 tablespoons minced dill
2 tablespoons caraway seeds
seasoned salt to taste
6 tablespoons mascarpone cheese
6 tablespoons grated Parmesan cheese

Melt butter in a medium-sized saucepan. Add leek and cauliflower and sauté for 3 minutes. Stir in *Chicken Stock* and stock cube. Cook over medium heat for ½ hour. Remove from heat. Cool. Place in food processor and blend. Add cream and blend 10 seconds more. Return to pan. Stir in fresh dill and caraway seeds. Warm to desired heat. Place in individual bowls. Top each with 1 tablespoon mascarpone and 1 tablespoon Parmesan. Serve hot.

TOTAL GRAMS 66.9
GRAMS PER SERVING 11.2

Salads

Chicken Salad Ham Rolls

4 servings

140 g cooked chicken, diced
4 tablespoons mayonnaise
4 tablespoons chopped parsley
4 tablespoon chopped celery leaves
1 teaspoon seasoned salt
6 black olives, diced
4 tablespoons finely chopped green pepper
8 slices boiled ham
lettuce leaves

Combine all ingredients except ham and lettuce. Spread mixture on ham slices and roll each one up, insert cocktail stick and place them seam side down on bed of lettuce leaves.

TOTAL GRAMS 6.8
GRAMS PER SERVING 1.7

Fresh Tuna and Avocado Salad

6 servings

1 large avocado, stoned, peeled and cubed
2 celery sticks, chopped
6 radishes, sliced
2 tablespoons lemon juice
2 tablespoons tarragon vinegar
½ small onion, chopped
¼ teaspoon cayenne pepper
seasoned salt to taste
675 g fresh tuna, grilled

Toss all ingredients together well, except fish. Divide into 6 portions.
  Cut fish in strips and place across top of each serving.
  Serve with *Dill Vinaigrette* (page 98).

TOTAL GRAMS 29.7
GRAMS PER SERVING 5.0

Coleslaw

6 125-ml servings

4 tablespoons Dijon mustard
4 tablespoons mayonnaise
1 teaspoon sugar substitute (optional)
1 tablespoon lemon juice
½ teaspoon salt
1 medium cabbage, shredded (about 225 g)

Mix mustard, mayonnaise, sugar substitute, lemon juice and salt
together. Add cabbage and toss well.

TOTAL GRAMS 41.4
GRAMS PER SERVING 6.9

Moulded Roquefort Spread

12 servings

1 tablespoon gelatine
60 ml cold water
180 g Roquefort cheese
180 g full fat soft (cream) cheese, softened
125 ml whipping cream
4 spring onions, finely chopped
2 tablespoons pine kernels
4 black olives, chopped
seasoned salt to taste

Sprinkle gelatine over water.

Push Roquefort cheese through strainer. Add cream cheese and cream to Roquefort cheese. Mix well. Add gelatine, spring onions, pine kernels, olives and salt to cheese mixture. Mix well.

Pour into 750 ml capacity ring mould that has been sprayed with oil or non-stick cooking spray. Chill until set.

TOTAL GRAMS 25.9
GRAMS PER SERVING 2.2

Mock Potato Salad

8 125-ml servings

1 medium swede
1 teaspoon sugar substitute (optional)
1 tablespoon lemon juice
60 g spring onions, finely chopped
1 medium dill pickle, chopped
120 g finely chopped celery with leaves
1½ teaspoon salt
dash of paprika
170 g mayonnaise
4 hard-boiled eggs, chopped

Pare swede, and cut into 4 pieces. Drop into boiling water and boil until tender, about ½ hour. Drain well. Cool.

After swede has cooled, dice and place in salad bowl. Sprinkle with sugar substitute, if using, and lemon juice. Add spring onions, pickle, celery, salt, paprika and mayonnaise.

Toss well. Fold in eggs. Chill before serving.

TOTAL GRAMS 48.0
GRAMS PER SERVING 6.0

Tossed Salad with Tomato Dressing

12 servings

2 heads lettuce (any variety)
2 tomatoes, peeled and deseeded
6 spring onions, finely chopped
1 tablespoon dry mustard
½ teaspoon garlic powder
1 tablespoon Dijon mustard
1 teaspoon seasoned salt
30 ml olive oil
30 ml tarragon vinegar
60 ml vegetable oil
1 tablespoon mayonnaise

Wash lettuce, dry thoroughly and tear into bite-size pieces. Refrigerate.

Tomato Dressing
Chop tomatoes and mash with spring onions until almost a paste. Add remaining ingredients except lettuce. Beat with wire whisk. Refrigerate.

When ready to serve, place lettuce in large salad bowl, pour dressing on top and toss well. Serve immediately.

TOTAL GRAMS 28.0
GRAMS PER SERVING 2.3

Not Just Another Tossed Salad

12 servings

900 g large prawns, peeled and deveined
125 ml garlic oil
225 g fresh spinach, washed and dried
1 small round lettuce, washed and dried
70 g large black olives,stoned and sliced
60 g diced celery
5 spring onions, chopped
6 radishes, sliced
70 g diced raw cauliflower florets
1 avocado, stoned, peeled and diced
8 rashers crispy cooked bacon, crumbled
2 soft-boiled eggs (2 minutes), peeled
125 ml lemon juice
60 ml groundnut oil
30 g grated Parmesan cheese
seasoned salt to taste

Sauté prawns in garlic oil until they turn pink. Refrigerate while you prepare salad.

Tear spinach and lettuce leaves into bite-size pieces. Toss all vegetables and bacon together in bowl.

Make dressing by beating eggs, lemon juice, oil, cheese and salt together.

Top salad with prawns. Pour dressing over salad and serve.

TOTAL GRAMS 65.0
GRAMS PER SERVING 5.4

Greek Salad

6 servings

1 large tomato, cubed
½ large green pepper, deseeded and cubed
½ large cucumber, pared and cubed
80 g stoned ripe olives
3 spring onions, chopped
2 tablespoons capers, drained
120 g feta cheese, crumbled
12 thin slices pepperoni
60 ml olive oil
30 ml wine vinegar
¼ teaspoon cracked pepper
½ teaspoon dried oregano

Combine tomato, pepper, cucumber, olives, spring onions, capers, cheese and pepperoni in salad bowl. Mix olive oil, vinegar, pepper and oregano together in small bowl. Pour dressing over vegetables. Toss and serve.

TOTAL GRAMS 28.9
GRAMS PER SERVING 4.8

Honeydew and Seafood

6 servings

1 450-g honeydew melon
1 180-g can tuna, drained
1 125-g can prawns, drained, or peeled small prawns
1 medium cucumber, peeled and cubed
225 g raw mushrooms, sliced
110 g mayonnaise
2 tablespoons passata, or tomato purée
½ teaspoon seasoned salt

Cut melon in half. Discard seeds and scoop out flesh, using a melon baller, or cube, leaving 1 cm on rinds. Cut each melon shell into thirds.

In bowl combine tuna, prawns (save a few for garnish), cucumber, mushrooms and melon balls.

Combine mayonnaise, passata, or tomato purée, and salt. Pour dressing over seafood mixture. Mix well.

Mound on melon shells. Garnish with some prawns.

If you prefer low fat, eliminate dressing and use juice of 1 lemon.

TOTAL GRAMS 47.0
GRAMS PER SERVING 7.8

Chicken Salad

2 servings

280 g cooked chicken meat, skinned and diced
60 g marinated artichoke hearts, drained
20 black olives, stoned
30 g finely chopped onion
15 g unsalted butter, melted
2 tablespoons crème fraîche or soured cream
1 tablespoon mayonnaise
seasoned salt to taste

Toss first 5 ingredients together. Mix crème fraîche and mayonnaise together. Add to chicken mixture. Mix well. Season with salt.

Refrigerate.

TOTAL GRAMS 8.4

GRAMS PER SERVING 4.2

Poached Salmon Salad

2 servings

whole leaves of 1 chicory
1 small tomato, peeled and quartered
1 small ripe avocado, stoned, peeled and diced
¼ small onion, diced (extra-sweet, if possible)
6 stoned black olives
2 salmon fillets, poached and cut into 2.5-cm strips
1 recipe Lime Dill Dressing *(page 91)*

Wash and dry chicory leaves. Chop tomato, avocado, onion and olives together in a wooden chopping bowl. Poach salmon and allow it to come to room temperature.

Place chicory leaves in a daisy formation in a round, shallow salad bowl. Put chopped tomato mixture the centre of the daisy. Place strips of salmon in each of the chicory leaves. Artistically dot with *Lime Dill Dressing*.

TOTAL GRAMS 19.8

GRAMS PER SERVING 9.9

Hot Beef Salad

6 servings

1 small round lettuce
1 small head Chinese leaves
1 large cucumber, sliced thin
1 red onion, peeled and sliced thin
½ small daikon radish, sliced thin
2 small tomatoes, cut in eight pieces
6 mint leaves
6 coriander leaves
60 ml walnut oil
675 g sirloin steak, sliced thin
½ teaspoon seasoned salt

Dressing:
5 garlic cloves, minced
60 ml fresh lime juice
1–2 teaspoons sugar substitute
1 tablespoon Tamari soy sauce
2 teaspoons crushed red pepper flakes
30 g mature Cheddar cheese, diced, for garnish

Wash and dry lettuce and Chinese leaves. Tear into bite-sized pieces. Mix onions, radishes, tomatoes, and mint and coriander leaves together and pour over lettuce. Toss.

Heat oil in a non-stick frying pan over medium heat. Add meat and seasoned salt. Cook quickly, stirring frequently, just until rare.

Artistically arrange cooked meat on salad. Mix dressing ingredients together and pour over salad. Top with Cheddar cubes.

TOTAL GRAMS 51.8
GRAMS PER SERVING 8.6

Leftover Lamb or Pork Salad

2 servings

450 g cooked leftover lamb or pork
seasoned salt to taste
pepper to taste
45 ml extra-virgin olive oil
2 tablespoons finely chopped fresh rosemary
15 ml balsamic vinegar
1 teaspoon Dijon mustard
2 heads little gem lettuce, cored, washed and dried
30 g Parmesan cheese shavings

Thinly slice lamb or pork. Whisk together salt, pepper, oil, rosemary, vinegar and mustard.

Place greens in a salad bowl with Parmesan shavings and toss them with the dressing. Arrange meat over greens.

TOTAL GRAMS 14.9
GRAMS PER SERVING 7.5

Salad Niçoise

12 servings

2 teaspoons Dijon mustard
30 ml wine vinegar
1½ teaspoons salt
2 cloves garlic, finely chopped
90 ml groundnut or vegetable oil
90 ml olive oil
freshly ground black pepper
1 teaspoon chopped thyme, or ½ teaspoon dried
900 g green beans
2 green peppers
4 celery sticks
280 g cherry tomatoes
3 × 200-g cans tuna, drained
1 60-g can anchovies, drained
10 stuffed green olives
10 black olives
1 large or 2 small red onions
2 tablespoons chopped basil, or 1 teaspoon dried
5 tablespoons finely chopped parsley
40 g finely chopped spring onions
6 hard-boiled eggs, quartered

Combine mustard, vinegar, salt, garlic, groundnut and olive oil, pepper and thyme in a bowl. Beat with a fork until well blended. Set aside.

Pick over beans and break into 3.5-cm lengths. Place beans in a saucepan and cook, in salted water to cover, until crisp-tender. Run under cold water and drain in a colander. Set aside.

Remove cores, seeds and white membranes from green peppers. Cut peppers in thin rounds. Set aside.

Trim celery sticks and cut crossways into thin slices. Set aside.

Use a large salad bowl and make a more or less symmetrical pattern of the green beans, peppers, celery and tomatoes. Flake the tuna and add to bowl. Arrange anchovies on top and scatter olives over all.

Peel onions and cut them into thin, almost transparent slices.

Scatter onion rings over all. Sprinkle with basil, parsley and spring onions. Serve with dressing. Garnish with eggs.

TOTAL GRAMS 116.0
GRAMS PER SERVING 9.7

Crunchy Seafood Salad

10 servings

1 × 180-g can tuna
1 × 180-g can crab meat
1 × 140-g can prawns, or cooked peeled prawns
1 large head lettuce
120 g diced celery
80 g chopped spring onions
½ medium ripe avocado, diced
50 g chopped walnuts
50 g roasted unsalted soybeans
50 g sunflower seeds
2 hard-boiled eggs, diced
1 tomato, cut in wedges

Drain the 3 cans of seafood; discard bony tissue from crab. Combine tuna and crab with prawns. Place in a bowl and refrigerate.

Combine remaining ingredients except tomato in a large salad bowl, and toss well.

Add seafood and toss again.

Add salad dressing of your choice.

Toss again before serving, and decorate with tomato wedges.

TOTAL GRAMS 74.8
GRAMS PER SERVING 7.5

Tricolor Salad with Three Cheeses

8 servings

1 recipe Mustard Vinaigrette *(page 92)*
1 small head of radicchio
3 chicory
1 head Cos lettuce or romaine
90 g Parmesan cheese shavings
150 g Camembert, cut into 8 wedges
120 g herby goat cheese, cut into 8 wedges
40 g pine kernels, toasted (or substitute Toasted Nuts*)*

Preheat oven to 230° C (gas 8).

Prepare vinaigrette and place in refrigerator for ½ hour. Separate leaves of lettuces. Wash and dry greens (make sure they are very dry), and tear into bite-size pieces.

Place in large salad bowl. Toss in Parmesan cheese.

Place Camembert and goat cheese wedges on a non-stick baking tray to melt in oven for 1 minute.

Place cheese wedges on salad. Top with dressing and pine kernels and serve.

TOTAL GRAMS 34.7
GRAMS PER SERVING 4.3

Salad Dressings

Mustard Vinaigrette

300 ml

1 teaspoon Dijon mustard
¼ teaspoon dry mustard
2 tablespoons finely chopped dill (or other herb)
15 ml balsamic vinegar
½ teaspoon seasoned salt
250 ml extra-virgin olive oil

Whisk ingredients together in a small bowl until well blended. Refrigerate for ½ hour.

TOTAL GRAMS 4.5
GRAMS PER TABLESPOON 0.2

Lime Dill Dressing (vinegar-free)

270 ml

250 ml extra-virgin olive oil
1 teaspoon Dijon mustard
¼ teaspoon dry mustard
juice of 1 lime
¼ teaspoon seasoned salt
1 clove garlic, finely chopped
1 tablespoon finely chopped dill
pinch sugar substitute

Whisk ingredients together in a small bowl. Refrigerate for ½ hour.

TOTAL GRAMS 3.0
GRAMS PER TABLESPOON 0.2

Tomato Mayonnaise (without vinegar)

300 ml

1 organic egg
1 teaspoon lemon juice
½ teaspoon seasoned salt
¼ teaspoon dried mustard
185 ml olive oil
1 small ripe tomato, peeled and deseeded
2 tablespoons finely chopped basil

Place first 4 ingredients in a food processor and blend. Add oil in a slow steady stream until it is fully blended. Chop tomato pulp and add to food processor with the basil. Blend for 30 seconds.

TOTAL GRAMS 5.9
GRAMS PER TABLESPOON 0.3

Basic Vinegar-Free Salad Dressing

240 ml

1 teaspoon seasoned salt
¼ teaspoon black pepper
1 teaspoon dry mustard
dash of Tabasco sauce
60 ml lemon juice
160 ml olive oil

Whisk all ingredients together. Refrigerate.

TOTAL GRAMS 7.0
GRAMS PER TABLESPOON 0.5

Vinegar-Free Mayonnaise

300 ml

1 organic egg
30 ml lemon juice
1 teaspoon Dijon mustard
¼ teaspoon dry mustard
¼ teaspoon seasoned salt
250 ml olive oil

Place first 5 ingredients in a blender. Drizzle oil into blender very slowly in a steady stream until it is fully blended.

TOTAL GRAMS 3.9
GRAMS PER TABLESPOON 0.2

Vinegar-Free Mustard

2 tablespoons (1 serving)

2 tablespoons Vinegar-Free Mayonnaise
¼ teaspoon dry mustard

Blend well. For more mustard flavour, increase dry mustard.

TOTAL GRAMS 0.5

Our Favourite Roquefort Dressing

240 ml

60 ml tarragon vinegar
¼ teaspoon seasoned salt
3 turns of pepper mill
90 ml olive oil
30 ml whipping cream
½ teaspoon lemon juice
30 g crumbled Roquefort cheese

Whisk all ingredients together except cheese. Stir in cheese.

TOTAL GRAMS 6.0
GRAMS PER TABLESPOON 0.4

Basic French Dressing

180 ml

45 ml tarragon vinegar
15 ml lemon juice
½ teaspoon seasoned salt
3 turns of pepper mill
90 ml olive oil
30 ml vegetable oil
½ teaspoon Dijon mustard
¼ teaspoon dry mustard

Whisk all ingredients together until well blended.

TOTAL GRAMS 4.7
GRAMS PER TABLESPOON 0.4

Vinaigrette Cream Dressing

480 ml

125 ml tarragon vinegar
¾ teaspoon salt
¼ teaspoon cracked pepper
375 ml olive oil (or 125 ml olive oil and 250 ml vegetable oil)
1 teaspoon chopped green olives
1 teaspoon chopped parsley
3 tablespoons soured cream
1 yolk from hard-boiled egg, finely chopped

Mix vinegar, salt and pepper. Add oil, olives, parsley, soured cream and chopped yolk.

Beat well with fork. Chill for several hours.

TOTAL GRAMS 9.3
GRAMS PER TABLESPOON 0.3

Dressing of the House

150 ml

30 ml olive oil
60 ml vegetable oil
30 ml tarragon vinegar
1 teaspoon seasoned salt
1 teaspoon Dijon mustard
¼ teaspoon garlic powder
1 tablespoon mayonnaise
¼ teaspoon sugar substitute

Put all ingredients in screw-top jar. Close jar and shake until well blended. Refrigerate.

TOTAL GRAMS 3.8
GRAMS PER TABLESPOON 0.4

Thousand Island Dressing

300 ml

6 spring onions
1 large dill pickle
2 tomatoes
½ teaspoon garlic powder
1 teaspoon seasoned salt
30 ml olive oil
30 ml tarragon vinegar
2 tablespoons mayonnaise

Chop spring onions, pickle and tomatoes together in wooden chopping bowl. Add rest of ingredients and mix well. Refrigerate.

TOTAL GRAMS 18.8
GRAMS PER TABLESPOON 0.9

Creamy Celery-Seed Dressing

285 ml

90 g soured cream
110 g mayonnaise
2 tablespoons passata or tomato purée
½ teaspoon Worcestershire sauce
½ teaspoon celery seed
½ teaspoon seasoned salt

Combine all ingredients in a screw-top jar. Shake well. Refrigerate.

TOTAL GRAMS 9.1
GRAMS PER TABLESPOON 0.5

Dill Vinaigrette Dressing

240 ml

60 ml tarragon vinegar
30 ml olive oil
90 ml sunflower oil
2 tablespoons chopped olives
¼ teaspoon dry mustard
1 teaspoon Dijon mustard
1 teaspoon lemon juice
¼ teaspoon garlic powder
3 tablespoons chopped fresh dill (or 2 teaspoons dried dill)
1 teaspoon sugar substitute
1 organic egg, beaten until frothy

Place all ingredients in a screw-top jar. Shake well. Refrigerate.

TOTAL GRAMS 9.0
GRAMS PER TABLESPOON 0.6

Curry Dressing

210 ml

60 ml tarragon vinegar
30 ml olive oil
90 ml sunflower oil
1 teaspoon lemon juice
½ teaspoon curry powder
1 tablespoon soured cream
¼ teaspoon garlic powder
1 teaspoon sesame seeds
½ teaspoon seasoned salt
1 organic egg, beaten until frothy

Place all ingredients in a screw-top jar. Shake well. Refrigerate.

TOTAL GRAMS 7.4
GRAMS PER TABLESPOON 0.5

Italian Dressing

210 ml

125 ml olive oil
60 ml wine vinegar
1 clove garlic, finely chopped
½ teaspoon seasoned salt
¼ teaspoon pepper

Combine all ingredients in a screw-top jar. Shake well. Refrigerate.
Shake again before serving.

TOTAL GRAMS 5.1
GRAMS PER TABLESPOON 0.4

Parmesan Caesar Dressing

210 ml

60 ml tarragon vinegar
30 ml olive oil
90 ml sunflower oil
1 teaspoon lemon juice
¼ teaspoon dry mustard
2 teaspoons Dijon mustard
1 tablespoon grated Parmesan cheese
¼ teaspoon garlic powder
1 teaspoon seasoned salt
1 teaspoon sugar substitute
1 organic egg, beaten until frothy

Place all ingredients in a screw-top jar. Shake well. Refrigerate.

TOTAL GRAMS 7.4
GRAMS PER TABLESPOON 0.5

Meat

Oriental Beef Stir Fry

4 servings

225 g spinach, steamed and drained
675 g beef fillet
90 ml spicy sesame oil
60 ml Tamari soy sauce
pepper to taste
225 g shiitake mushrooms, sliced thin
1 onion, sliced thin
125 g bamboo shoots, cut into thin strips
3 celery sticks, cut into thin strips
2 tablespoons sake
125 ml Beef Stock *(page 71)*

Drain spinach well. Cut meat into thin strips and sauté in a large frying pan using half of the sesame oil. Brown meat on both sides. Sprinkle with 30 ml of the soy sauce and pepper. Remove meat from pan. Put mushrooms, onion, bamboo shoots and celery into frying pan with remaining oil. Sauté for 3 minutes. Return beef to pan, add spinach and toss with remaining soy sauce, sake and stock. Cook over low heat for 6–8 minutes or to preferred doneness.

TOTAL GRAMS 37.2
GRAMS PER SERVING   9.3

Kayzie's Rabbit

6 servings

1½–2 kg rabbit, jointed
250 ml olive oil, plus more for sprinkling
juice of 1 large lemon
½ teaspoon rosemary
½ teaspoon fennel seeds
½ teaspoon seasoned salt
8 cloves garlic, finely chopped
1 large onion, sliced thin
4 small carrots, sliced thin
2 bay leaves
125 g thick-sliced streaky bacon
100 g shiitake mushrooms, sliced
500 ml Chicken Stock *(page 69)*

Wash and dry rabbit.

Mix 125 ml of the olive oil, lemon juice, rosemary, fennel, salt and garlic in a large bowl. Add onions and carrots.

Spread half of vegetable mixture on bottom of a shallow glass dish. Place rabbit pieces on top. Top with remaining vegetable mixture. Place bay leaves on top. Cover dish and place in refrigerator for 2 days. Sprinkle with olive oil daily.

To cook:

Remove rabbit from vegetable mixture, and save the vegetables.

Slice bacon into bite-size pieces and brown in a large casserole or deep frying pan. Add the remaining 125 ml olive oil to frying pan and brown rabbit pieces well on all sides. Remove and set aside.

Drain vegetable mixture. Place vegetables in still hot pan and lightly brown. Add rabbit back to pan, cover with *Chicken Stock,* heat to a simmer. Cover and cook for 1½ hours, or until very tender.

TOTAL GRAMS 58.4
GRAMS PER SERVING 9.7

Mother's Pot Roast

6 servings

1.7 kg top rump of beef
½ teaspoon garlic powder
1 teaspoon seasoned salt
2 medium onions, sliced
2 cloves of garlic
3 tomatoes, skinned and quartered

Rub garlic powder and seasoned salt into the meat. Place in refrigerator for ½ hour.

Place onions and garlic in a food processor. Push tomatoes through a sieve to rid them of seeds and place tomato pulp in food processor. Purée.

Place meat in a large pot or casserole. Cover with puréed tomatoes, add water if needed, cover the pot and simmer for 1½ hours. Turn meat and simmer about 1½ hours more or until fork-soft. Remove meat from pot to a cutting board to cool. Place sauce in refrigerator to allow fat to rise to top. When meat is cool, slice. Remove fat that has formed on the sauce and place meat back in the sauce. Warm and serve.

TOTAL GRAMS 35.5
GRAMS PER SERVING 5.9

THE HAMBURGERS

Dr. Atkins Fromage Burger

6 servings

900 g minced beef
1 tablespoon chopped chives
1 tablespoon chopped tarragon (or ³/₄ teaspoon crushed dried tarragon)
2 teaspoons seasoned salt
10 g parsley, chopped
30 g spring onions, finely chopped
1 small tomato, diced
1 egg, beaten
185 g Cheddar cheese, coarsely grated
40 g butter (optional)

Combine beef, chives, tarragon, salt, parsley, spring onions, tomato and egg. Mix well.

Shape into 12 equal balls. Flatten each ball to a thin disc. Divide cheese into 6 piles. Press cheese together. Place 1 pile of cheese in the centre of 6 of the meat discs. Place second burger disc on top. Press edges together to seal.

Dr. Atkins likes to cook these on an outdoor barbecue. If one is not available, grill or sauté in butter in a non-stick frying pan for five minutes on each side.

TOTAL GRAMS 12.3
GRAMS PER SERVING 2.1

Brit Burgers

2 servings

60 g butter
60 g onion, chopped
450 g minced beef
½ teaspoon seasoned salt
½ teaspoon pepper
½ teaspoon sage

Melt half the butter in a frying pan. Sauté onions until golden. Remove and set aside.

Combine beef, salt, pepper and sage with onions and mix well. Shape into patties. In same pan melt remaining butter. Sauté for 5 minutes on each side.

TOTAL GRAMS 7.3
GRAMS PER SERVING 3.6

Pizza Burgers

6 servings

900 g minced beef
1 teaspoon seasoned salt
1 tablespoon chopped parsley
⅛ teaspoon dried basil
⅛ teaspoon dried oregano
2 eggs, beaten
1 package (50 g) fried pork rinds, crushed
60 ml olive oil
6 slices mozzarella cheese
½ recipe Pasta Sauce *(pages 182–3)*
20 g grated Parmesan cheese

Preheat oven to 200° C (gas 6).

Mix beef with salt, parsley, basil and oregano.

Shape into 6 patties 1-cm thick.

Dip patties into eggs, then coat with crushed pork rinds. Sauté patties in hot olive oil until well browned on both sides. Arrange in a shallow baking dish. They must not be touching. Top each patty with a slice of mozzarella cheese. Pour on *Pasta Sauce*. Sprinkle with Parmesan cheese. Bake for 15 minutes.

TOTAL GRAMS 66.2
GRAMS PER SERVING 11.0

Feta Burgers

2 servings

30 g butter
450 g minced beef
30 g crumbled feta cheese
4 tablespoons finely chopped black olives
½ teaspoon seasoned salt
½ teaspoon pepper

Melt butter in a heavy frying pan.
    Mix remaining ingredients and shape into patties.
    Sauté hamburgers for 5 minutes on each side.

TOTAL GRAMS 3.4
GRAMS PER SERVING 1.7

Curry Burgers

2 servings

30 g butter
450 g minced beef
1 tablespoon finely chopped walnuts
2 teaspoons curry powder
½ teaspoon seasoned salt

Melt butter in frying pan.
    Mix remainder of ingredients and shape into patties.
    Sauté hamburgers for 5 minutes on each side.

TOTAL GRAMS 3.6
GRAMS PER SERVING 1.8

¡Ole! Burgers

2 servings

2 tablespoons butter
450 g minced beef
6 drops Tabasco sauce
½ teaspoon cumin
½ teaspoon chilli powder
¼ teaspoon garlic powder

Melt butter in a frying pan.
    Mix remainder of ingredients and shape into patties.
    Sauté hamburgers for 5 minutes on each side.

TOTAL GRAMS 1.7
GRAMS PER SERVING 0.9

U.S. Hamburgers

2 servings

6 rashers lean streaky bacon
1 ripe tomato, finely chopped
2 tablespoons butter
450 g minced beef
½ teaspoon seasoned salt
½ teaspoon pepper

Fry bacon until crisp. Remove from frying pan, and place on kitchen paper to drain. Crumble bacon into a large bowl. Sauté tomato in bacon fat until tender. Add it to the bacon. Pour off bacon fat and melt butter in same pan. Combine meat, salt and pepper with bacon and tomato.

Shape into patties.

Sauté hamburgers for 5 minutes on each side.

TOTAL GRAMS 6.7
GRAMS PER SERVING 3.4

Steak Au Poivre

4 servings

4 sirloin steaks, pounded to 3-mm thickness
freshly ground black pepper
90 g butter
2 teaspoons chopped rosemary leaves
2 teaspoons chopped sage leaves
125 ml cognac, warmed
185 ml whipping cream
2 teaspoons Worcestershire sauce
2 tablespoons Dijon mustard

Cover surface of steaks on both sides with ground pepper.

Press pepper into steaks.

In a large frying pan melt butter and add rosemary and sage.

Add steaks and brown quickly on both sides. Pour warm cognac over steaks and ignite. When flame goes out, remove steaks from frying pan and keep warm.

Add cream, Worcestershire sauce and mustard to pan juices. Stir well and simmer for 3 minutes. Pour over steak and serve.

TOTAL GRAMS 14.2
GRAMS PER SERVING 3.6

Moussaka

6 servings

40 g unsalted butter
3 egg yolks
300 ml water
60 ml whipping cream
50 g grated Parmesan cheese
1 medium aubergine
450 g minced lamb or 225 g minced lean beef
90 ml olive oil
1 large onion, chopped
1 large green pepper, chopped
2 cloves garlic, minced
250 ml prepared tomato sauce or passata
1½ teaspoons ground cumin
¼ teaspoon grated nutmeg
¼ teaspoon dried oregano
2 teaspoons salt

Preheat oven to 180° C (gas 4).

To prepare cream sauce:
Place butter in top of double boiler over hot water. Add egg yolks one at a time. Beat constantly with rotary or hand electric beater. Add 60 ml of the water, cream and Parmesan cheese. Continue to beat until sauce thickens, about 10 minutes.

Pare and slice aubergine. Arrange aubergine on a large plate. Place plate in sink. Cover with another large plate, allowing plate to press aubergine. Let drain for ½ hour, then press each slice with kitchen paper. Heat 30 ml of the olive oil in a large frying pan. Add onion and green pepper. Sauté until light golden brown. Add garlic and meat, and cook until browned.

Add tomato sauce, remaining water, cumin, nutmeg, oregano and salt. Simmer for 15 minutes.

Heat remaining olive oil, and sauté aubergine slices until lightly browned. Drain on kitchen paper. Place half the aubergine slices in a well-oiled baking dish. Spread with half the meat mixture. Place remaining aubergine slices on top and cover with the rest of the meat. Cover top with cream sauce.

Bake for 30 minutes.

TOTAL GRAMS 68.7
GRAMS PER SERVING 11.5

Calf's Liver in Red Wine

4 servings

6 shallots or 1 small onion, finely chopped
250 ml dry red wine
juice of 1 lemon
60 ml oil
½ teaspoon dried oregano
½ teaspoon seasoned salt
¼ teaspoon black pepper
450 g calf's liver, sliced
60 g butter

Combine shallots, wine, lemon juice, oil, oregano, salt and pepper in a large bowl. Marinate liver for 1 hour, then turn it and marinate for another hour.

Remove liver from marinade.

Melt butter in a frying pan, and sauté liver for 5 minutes on each side.

TOTAL GRAMS 20.9
GRAMS PER SERVING 5.2

Veal Rolatine

4 servings

4 veal escalopes, flattened with a mallet
½ teaspoon seasoned salt
4 slices prosciutto ham
6 slices Jarlsberg cheese
1 egg, beaten
25 g grated Parmesan cheese
60 g unsalted butter
60 ml dry white wine

Preheat oven to 180° C (gas 4).

Rinse and dry veal. Sprinkle with salt. Place 1 slice of ham and 1 slice of cheese on each cutlet. Roll up and tie with string. Dip rolls in egg and coat with Parmesan cheese. Place in refrigerator for ½ hour to set. Melt butter in a heavy frying pan. Sauté veal rolls until they are brown on all sides. Remove rolls to a small baking dish. Add wine to pan juices and bring to a boil. Pour sauce over rolls. Top with 2 remaining slices of cheese. Bake for ½ hour. Remove string and serve.

Note: This may be used as an hors d'oeuvre by cutting rolls into bite-size pieces.

TOTAL GRAMS 4.1
GRAMS PER SERVING 1.0

Gourmet Pork Chops

6 servings

12 pork chops
salt and pepper to taste
30 ml garlic oil
30 ml olive oil
1 onion, chopped
1 clove garlic, minced
450 g mushrooms, sliced
250 ml hot Chicken Stock *(page 69)*
125 ml dry red wine
1 bay leaf
4 tablespoons soured cream (optional)

Preheat oven to 180° C (gas 4).

Sprinkle pork chops with salt and pepper. In a heavy frying pan brown chops in garlic oil over high heat. Remove and keep warm. Add olive oil to pan. Sauté onion, garlic and mushrooms in olive oil until onion is golden. Pour in *Chicken Stock* and wine, and add bay leaf. Bring mixture to a boil and cook for about 3 minutes.

Arrange 6 pork chops in casserole. Top with half the sauce.

Put another layer of pork chops on top and pour over remaining mixture. Cover casserole tightly and bake for 1½ hours.

If wished, soured cream may be added to sauce mixture when served.

TOTAL GRAMS 36.9
GRAMS PER SERVING 6.2

Roast Veal

6 servings

1 2–2.5 kg veal roast (leg, loin, rump, shoulder, or breast)
1 clove garlic, cut in slivers
225 g thick-sliced bacon (streaky or back)
3 tablespoons olive oil
40 g onion, chopped
2 celery sticks, diced
4 anchovies (optional)
125 ml white wine or Chicken Stock *(page 69)*

Preheat oven to 170° C (gas 3).

Have the butcher bone and tie meat. Cut a few incisions in veal and insert garlic.

In roasting tin with cover, or casserole, heat oil and brown veal. Add onion, celery, anchovies if using, and wine or stock to pan. Arrange bacon on top. Place in oven. Cover and cook for 30 minutes per 500 g, basting occasionally. Remove veal from pan, and let it rest for 10 minutes for easier carving. Remove vegetables from pan juices, skim off excess fat, and pour pan juices over veal. Serve warm, or serve cold, sliced with *Vinaigrette Cream Dressing,* page 96.

TOTAL GRAMS 7.9
GRAMS PER SERVING 1.3

Veal Scaloppini

6 servings

675 g veal cut in escalopes 5-mm thick
salt and pepper to taste
90 g butter
60 ml brandy
250 ml Chicken Stock *(page 69)*
60 ml Chablis, or other dry white wine
30 ml dry sherry
450 g porcini mushrooms, sliced
2 tomatoes, peeled and chopped
1 teaspoon garlic powder
60 g grated Swiss cheese
25 g grated Parmesan cheese

Preheat grill.

Pat salt and pepper into veal.

In a frying pan melt 50 g of the butter, then add veal to brown.

Heat brandy. Pour over veal and ignite. Remove veal from frying pan and keep warm. Pour *Chicken Stock,* Chablis and sherry into pan. Simmer until liquid reduces by half. Return veal to pan. Simmer for 10 minutes. Keep warm until serving.

Sauté mushrooms in remaining butter until brown. Add tomatoes and garlic powder. Simmer for 5 minutes. Place mushroom mixture in baking dish. Add veal and cover with wine sauce. Sprinkle with grated Swiss and Parmesan cheeses.

Grill until cheese is brown and bubbly. Serve immediately.

TOTAL GRAMS 38.9
GRAMS PER SERVING   6.5

My Grandmother's Veal Stew

4 servings

3 rashers back bacon, diced
40 g butter
1 tablespoon chopped onion
40 g mushrooms, sliced
900 g cubed stewing veal
125 ml water or Chicken Stock *(page 69)*
225 g soured cream
1 teaspoon salt
¼ teaspoon paprika

Preheat oven to 120° C (gas ³/₄).

Place bacon, butter, onion and mushrooms in frying pan. Sauté slowly until onion and bacon are lightly brown. Remove mixture with slotted spoon. Place in ovenproof serving dish. Leave bacon fat and butter in frying pan, then add veal. Brown meat on all sides. Remove veal, leaving fat in pan. Place meat in baking dish. Mix well with bacon mixture.

Add water or stock, soured cream, salt and paprika to fat in frying pan. Heat just to boiling. Pour over meat mixture. Cover dish. Bake for 1 hour, or until veal is tender when pierced with fork.

TOTAL GRAMS 12.0
GRAMS PER SERVING 3.0

Garden Beef

8 servings

60 ml vegetable oil
1.4 kg stewing steak (chuck or topside), cubed
40 g onion, chopped
1 litre water
3 soup bones
2 teaspoons salt
100 g swede, cubed
½ medium green pepper, chopped
¼ small aubergine, chopped
60 g courgette, cubed
60 ml prepared tomato sauce or passata
50 g spinach

Heat oil in large heavy pot. Add meat and brown well on all sides. Push meat to one side of pot and add onion. Cook 2 more minutes.

Add water, soup bones and salt. Simmer for 2 hours.

Add swede and simmer for 15 more minutes.

Add green pepper, aubergine and courgette. Simmer for 10 more minutes. Spoon in tomato sauce or passata and spinach, and cook for 7 more minutes.

TOTAL GRAMS 20.8
GRAMS PER SERVING 2.6

Luscious Lamb

4 servings

8 lamb chops
garlic powder
30 g butter
30 ml Worcestershire sauce
30 ml lemon juice
30 ml gin
1 teaspoon seasoned salt

Rub lamb chops with small amount of garlic powder and place in a dish. Melt butter in a small pan and add Worcestershire sauce, lemon juice, gin and salt. Pour liquid over lamb chops. Allow to marinate in refrigerator for 30 minutes. Remove lamb from marinade. Grill or barbecue to desired doneness. Meanwhile, boil marinade in a small saucepan for 10 minutes. Top lamb with marinade before serving.

TOTAL GRAMS 9.9
GRAMS PER SERVING 2.5

Stuffed Leg of Lamb

8 servings

30 g butter
450 g minced veal or beef
30 g chopped onion
1 clove garlic, minced
125 ml white wine
250 ml prepared tomato sauce or passata
1 tablespoon chopped dill
1 tablespoon chopped parsley
50 g grated Parmesan cheese
salt and pepper to taste
1 leg of lamb, boned and flattened

Preheat oven to 150° C (gas 2).
    Melt half the butter in heavy frying pan. Add minced meat, onion

and garlic. Brown lightly on all sides. Pour wine in pan slowly, and cook for 2 minutes. Add tomato sauce or passata, dill and parsley. Cook over medium heat for 10 minutes, or until liquid has been absorbed. Remove from heat. Sprinkle with Parmesan cheese, salt and pepper. Wipe lamb with damp cloth. Sprinkle with salt and pepper.

Spread minced meat mixture on lamb and roll up carefully. Use skewers to fasten it or tie with string.

Melt remaining butter in medium-size roasting tin. Add lamb roll. Brown over medium heat.

Bake for 2 hours or until meat is tender. (If the pan gets dry, add 2 or 3 tablespoons water to tin.)

TOTAL GRAMS 25.3
GRAMS PER SERVING 3.2

Loin of Lamb with Horseradish Cream

6 servings

2 × 1.4 kg lamb loins, boned and trimmed of fat, bones reserved
3 bay leaves
3 celery sticks, chopped
6 black peppercorns
1 litre water
1 clove garlic, quartered
1 onion, chopped
60 ml walnut oil
salt and freshly ground pepper to taste
500 ml whipping cream
3 tablespoons grated white horseradish, drained
2 tablespoons snipped chives

Place lamb bones, bay leaf, celery and peppercorns in the water. Bring water to a boil, skimming off foam, and simmer mixture until liquid is reduced to about 625 ml. Strain stock through a fine sieve into a pan. Add garlic and onions. Bring liquid to a boil. Simmer until it is reduced to 375 ml. Strain the stock.

In a large frying pan, heat oil over medium heat until it is hot (do not allow it to smoke). Season lamb with salt and pepper and brown in oil. Turn lamb to brown well on all sides. Remove lamb from oil, cool for 10 minutes, and slice it 1-cm thick. Arrange slices on a platter and keep warm. Return stock to frying pan, and stir in cream and horseradish. Gently simmer sauce until it thickens (do not boil). Adjust seasonings and spoon over lamb. Garnish with chives.

TOTAL GRAMS 29.2
GRAMS PER SERVING 4.9

Steak Pizzaiola

6 servings

30 ml garlic oil
60 ml olive oil
30 ml tarragon vinegar
1 teaspoon water
freshly cracked black pepper
1.4 kg sirloin steak
8 Italian plum tomatoes, cut into strips
2 cloves garlic, crushed
1 tablespoon chopped parsley
1 teaspoon dried oregano
⅛ teaspoon seasoned salt
40 g pine kernels
1 teaspoon sugar substitute (optional)

Combine garlic oil with half the olive oil, the vinegar, water and pepper. Place steak in mixture and marinate in refrigerator for at least 2 hours, preferably overnight. Heat remaining olive oil, and add tomatoes, garlic, parsley, oregano, salt and pine kernels. Cook over medium heat for 3 minutes. Remove from heat, add sugar substitute if using, and keep warm. Grill steak to preferred doneness, slice, and pour mixture over it. Serve immediately.

TOTAL GRAMS 21.9
GRAMS PER SERVING 3.7

Cabbage Rolls Stuffed with Meat (Dolma)

6 servings

1 medium cabbage
675 g minced lamb or beef
40 g diced onion
4 tablespoons chopped parsley
2 eggs
1 teaspoon salt
pepper to taste
80 ml prepared tomato sauce or passata

Sauce:
70 g chopped cabbage
125 ml water
160 ml prepared tomato sauce or passata
2 tablespoons lemon juice
1 tablespoon sugar substitute

Clean cabbage and remove any damaged leaves. Pour boiling water over cabbage. Cover and let stand for ½ hour. Mix minced meat, onion, parsley, eggs, salt, pepper and passata together.

Drain cabbage, core, and separate leaves.

To stuff:
Use 12 leaves. Put 3 full tablespoons of meat mixture in centre of each leaf. Bring sides up over filling and roll leaf up. Set aside.

Sauce:
Chop remaining cabbage (the core and leaves not suitable for stuffing). Heat water in medium-size pot. Bring to boil. Add chopped cabbage, tomato sauce or passata, salt, lemon juice and sugar substitute. Reduce heat, cover, and simmer for 15 minutes.

Remove 250 ml sauce and set aside. Place cabbage rolls in pot with remaining sauce as close together as possible. Pour reserved sauce over cabbage rolls. Cover. Simmer for 1½ hours.

TOTAL GRAMS 61.6
GRAMS PER SERVING 10.2

Spicy Spare Ribs

4 servings

1.8 kg pork spare ribs, or beef ribs
1 tablespoon paprika
2 teaspoons chilli powder
¾ teaspoon salt
½ teaspoon dry mustard
¼ teaspoon garlic powder
⅛ teaspoon pepper

Preheat oven to 230° C (gas 8).

Place single layer of ribs, meaty side down, in shallow roasting tin. Roast for ½ hour. Drain off fat. Combine rest of ingredients, sprinkle evenly over ribs.

Reduce oven to 180° C (gas 4). Roast, meaty side up, for a further ½–1 hour for spare ribs. Beef ribs will take about 1 hour longer.

TOTAL GRAMS 7.2
GRAMS PER SERVING 1.8

Stuffed Steak

6 servings

1.4 kg of any thick cut of steak
garlic powder
225 g shiitake mushrooms
½ teaspoon thyme
3 sprigs parsley, chopped
5 slices smoked ham
30 g unsalted butter
2 shallots or 1 small onion, finely chopped
1 clove garlic, chopped
30 ml dry white wine

Using a sharp knife, make a pocket in the steak. Rub garlic powder on steak and set aside.

Chop together mushrooms, thyme, parsley and ham in large wooden chopping bowl.

Heat butter over low flame until melted. Brown shallots and garlic in butter. Add mushroom mixture and cook for 3 minutes, stirring occasionally. Add wine and cook 1 more minute. Remove from heat and spoon mushroom mixture into pockets in steak. Stuff firmly, and sew closed with a trussing needle and thread.

Grill steak to preferred doneness.

Serve with hot *Parsley Butter Sauce,* page 186.

TOTAL GRAMS 17.5
GRAMS PER SERVING 2.9

Pork Loin with Mustard

6 servings

6 1-cm slices of boneless pork loin
salt and freshly ground black pepper
30 ml olive oil
20 g shallots, chopped
60 ml dry white wine
10 ml brandy
185 ml Chicken Stock *(page 69)*
1 tablespoon sugar substitute
1 tablespoon Dijon mustard

Season pork well with salt and pepper.

Heat oil in a large frying pan over medium heat. Do not allow it to smoke. Brown pork in oil. Remove pork, lower heat, and add shallots. Cook them for about 3 minutes. Pour in wine and brandy and simmer until liquid has evaporated. Add stock and sugar substitute. Whisk mixture as it boils until liquid is reduced by half. Add pork and simmer for about 2 minutes until pork is warm and has absorbed some sauce. Remove pork to a serving plate. Whisk mustard into sauce, correct seasonings, and spoon remaining sauce over pork.

TOTAL GRAMS 7.2
GRAMS PER SERVING 1.2

Poultry

Chicken Cacciatore

8 servings

1 2.2 kg chicken, jointed into 8 pieces
125 ml olive oil
60 g butter
60 g chopped onion
225 g shiitake mushrooms, sliced
3 cloves garlic
185 ml dry white wine
2 bay leaves
1 teaspoon basil
½ teaspoon freshly ground black pepper
75 ml prepared tomato sauce or passata
seasoned salt to taste
2 tablespoons brandy

In a large frying pan, sauté chicken in olive oil until light golden brown, about 20 minutes.

Heat butter in a separate frying pan until melted; add onion and mushrooms and sauté until golden. Add garlic. Cook for 4 more minutes. Spoon mushrooms, onions and garlic over chicken. Pour on wine. Add bay leaves, basil and pepper. Simmer for about 8 minutes, uncovered. Stir in tomato sauce or passata. Salt to taste. Cook, uncovered, over low heat for 15 more minutes. Add brandy, and serve.

TOTAL GRAMS 31.1
GRAMS PER SERVING 3.8

Lemon-Basted Roast Chicken

4 servings

4 chicken portions (legs or breasts with wings)
½ teaspoon dried oregano
¼ teaspoon garlic powder
60 g butter
salt and pepper to taste
juice of 2 lemons (6 to 8 tablespoons)

Preheat oven to 200° C (gas 6).

Sprinkle chicken with oregano and garlic powder. Melt butter in roasting tin or casserole. Add chicken; turn to coat. Sprinkle with salt and pepper.

Roast chicken skin-side up, uncovered, for 30 minutes or until golden brown. Turn pieces over and continue roasting until brown, about 30 more minutes. Reduce heat to 150° C (gas 2) and cook until tender. Squeeze lemon juice over chicken.

Cover and let rest in turned-off oven for 15 minutes.

Remove to platter and serve.

TOTAL GRAMS 6.2
GRAMS PER SERVING 1.6

Coq Au Vin with Shiitake Mushrooms

8 servings

4 rashers thick-sliced bacon
100 g butter
1 × 1.8 kg chicken, jointed into 8 pieces
1 teaspoon seasoned salt
60 ml cognac (or brandy)
250 ml dry red wine
250 ml Chicken Stock *(page 69)*
¼ teaspoon garlic powder
¾ teaspoon thyme
1 bay leaf
4 medium-size onions, sliced
225 g shiitake mushrooms, sliced
chopped chives

Dice bacon and sauté in 60 g of the butter in large frying pan until brown. Remove bacon from pan and reserve.

Rinse and thoroughly dry chicken. Brown in bacon fat and season with salt.

Put bacon back in pan, cover, and simmer for about 10 minutes.

Heat cognac in small pan. Ignite, and pour over chicken. Add wine, stock, garlic powder and thyme. Add bay leaf to chicken, cover and simmer for 45 minutes. Remove chicken and keep warm.

Boil liquid in pan until it reduces by half.

In a separate pan, sauté onions and mushrooms in remaining butter until onions are golden.

Put chicken back into frying pan. Cover with mushrooms and onions. Simmer for 5 minutes. Garnish with chives.

TOTAL GRAMS 39.8
GRAMS PER SERVING 5.0

Chicken à la Firenze

4 servings

4 chicken breast fillets
2 eggs, beaten
25 g fried pork rinds, crushed
45 g butter
125 ml Sauterne
250 ml Chicken Stock *(page 69)*
1 clove garlic, finely chopped
pinch of dried marjoram
pinch of dried basil
80 ml whipping cream
225 g spinach, cooked*
30 g grated Parmesan cheese

Preheat oven to 180° C (gas 4).

Dip chicken in eggs and dredge in crushed pork rinds until well coated. Sauté in butter until chicken begins to brown. Turn once. Lower heat. Add wine and cook until wine has almost evaporated. Remove chicken breasts and reserve.

Mix together stock, garlic, marjoram, basil and cream. Pour into pan and heat with pan juices.

Place half the spinach in bottom of casserole. Add chicken; top with remaining spinach. Pour sauce over top. Sprinkle with Parmesan cheese and bake for ½ hour.

TOTAL GRAMS 16.5
GRAMS PER SERVING 4.1

---

*To cook fresh spinach: Wash carefully several times to remove all sand. Place in pot with just enough water to cover it. Cook at low boil for about 10 minutes or until tender, but not limp. Press out water before serving. Two packages of frozen spinach may be substituted for fresh spinach. Cook to package directions. Whether fresh or frozen do not overcook.

Summer Day Chicken From Spain

4 servings

1 2.2 kg chicken, jointed into pieces
60 ml sunflower oil
2 cloves garlic
juice of 1 lemon
1 teaspoon grated orange zest
2 bay leaves
125 ml vinegar
250 ml white wine
250 ml Chicken Stock *(page 69)*
½ teaspoon coarsely ground pepper
salt to taste

Rinse and dry chicken. Heat oil in frying pan. Lightly brown chicken over medium heat.

Combine remaining ingredients. Pour over chicken. Simmer, covered, for 1 hour. Add more stock, if necessary, to keep chicken covered.

Serve warm or chilled.

TOTAL GRAMS 18.6
GRAMS PER SERVING 4.7

Austrian Paprika Chicken

6 servings

30 g butter
30 ml vegetable oil
2 chickens, jointed, about 2.2 kg
seasoned salt
4 small onions, quartered
1 clove garlic, finely chopped
2 tablespoons paprika
250 ml Chicken Stock *(page 69)*
230 g soured cream

Preheat oven to 180° C (gas 4).

Heat butter and oil together. Brown chicken carefully in oil on all sides. Add salt. Remove chicken from pan.

Place onions and garlic in oil and sauté until onions are golden. Add paprika, stock and soured cream. Stir constantly until mixture is smooth.

Place chicken in casserole and cover with mixture, making sure to scrape pan well of all drippings.

Bake, covered, for 1 hour.

Serve with *Tossed Salad with Tomato Dressing,* page 82.

TOTAL GRAMS 34.8
GRAMS PER SERVING 5.8

Chicken Croquettes

2 servings

350 g minced chicken
2 egg whites
¼ teaspoon poultry seasoning (or pinch each ground nutmeg and
allspice)
pinch of salt
rapeseed or groundnut oil, for deep frying
20 g chopped onion
4 large mushrooms, chopped
15 g butter
Cream Sauce *(page 180)*

Preheat oven to 190° C (gas 5).

Mix chicken, egg whites, poultry seasoning and salt. Form into cylinders or croquettes 2.5 cm wide and 7.5 cm long. Fry in oil until crisp.

Sauté onion and mushrooms in butter until lightly browned.

Prepare *Cream Sauce*.

Place mushrooms and onion in a casserole and arrange croquettes on top.

Pour sauce on top.

Bake for about 8–10 minutes until thoroughly heated.

To make a prettier dish, place sliced hard-boiled eggs between croquettes. Then add sauce. Sprinkle with paprika.

TOTAL GRAMS 7.4
GRAMS PER SERVING 3.7

Gourmet Poussins

6 servings

170 g butter
185 ml white port wine
3 tablespoons dried tarragon
6 garlic cloves
1½ teaspoons salt
¾ teaspoon pepper
garlic powder
6 poussins, about 550 g each

Preheat oven to 200° C (gas 6).

Melt butter in a saucepan. Add wine and 1 tablespoon dried tarragon. Heat thoroughly.

Place 1 garlic clove, 1 teaspoon tarragon, ¼ teaspoon salt and ⅛ teaspoon pepper in each poussin. Sprinkle outside liberally with garlic powder.

Pour wine sauce over poussins and roast in large shallow tin, without rack, for about 1 hour, or until well browned and drumstick twists easily. Baste frequently with sauce.

TOTAL GRAMS 16.8
GRAMS PER SERVING 2.8

Turkey à la King

4 servings

4 egg yolks
¼ teaspoon seasoned salt
½ teaspoon dried tarragon
250 ml whipping cream
250 ml Chicken Stock (page 69)
280 g diced turkey meat
nutmeg

Preheat oven to 180° C (gas 4).

Whisk yolks until thick and lemon-coloured. Add salt and tarragon. Whisk in cream. Stir in stock, then add turkey meat.

Pour into 4 small ovenproof bowls. Sprinkle with nutmeg. Set bowls in shallow pan half-filled with water, and bake for 30 minutes.

TOTAL GRAMS 9.4
GRAMS PER SERVING 2.4

Roast Turkey

Preheat oven to 200° C (gas 6).

This is an easy, delicious way to cook a perfect, moist turkey. Have turkey at room temperature. Remove giblets from cavity. Run turkey under cold water to rinse inside and out. Never soak a turkey in water. Dry turkey well. Rub turkey with garlic inside and out. Place sliced oranges and lemons in the cavity if you are not stuffing it, or use the *Almond Stuffing* that follows. Insert poultry pins to draw open cavity together. Use string to lace between pins as you would lace a boot.

Tie legs together with string if not already tucked under a piece of string or skin. Bend wing tips under body and tuck loose neck skin under turkey.

Place turkey, breast side up, in a stainless-steel roasting tin that has a cover. Cover turkey breast with slices of turkey bacon. Place cover on pan.

Bake at 200° C (gas 6) for 20 minutes. Reduce to 180° C (gas 4). Cook for 20 minutes per 500 g if turkey is over 4.5 kg. If under 4.5 kg, cook for 15 minutes per pound.

TOTAL GRAMS 0

Almond Stuffing

6 servings

120 g butter
80 g finely chopped onion
225 g smoked ham, chopped fine
10 g chopped parsley
½ teaspoon dried thyme, or 1 tablespoon fresh
½ teaspoon freshly ground pepper
40 g fried pork rinds, crushed
2 eggs
60 ml dry red wine
85 g blanched almonds

Melt butter in large frying pan. Add onions. Cook until light brown. Add ham, parsley and spices. Mix well. Combine mixture with pork rinds, eggs, wine and almonds.

Use to stuff chicken, turkey, veal roast, or anything that needs a stuffing.

TOTAL GRAMS 24.5
GRAMS PER SERVING   4.1

Duck in Red Wine

4 servings

30 g butter, or rendered duck or chicken fat
1 2.2–2.6 kg duck, skin removed, jointed into 8 pieces
2 cloves garlic, minced
500 ml dry red wine
8 shiitake mushrooms, thinly sliced
2 sprigs parsley, chopped
1 small bay leaf
¼ teaspoon dried thyme
1 teaspoon seasoned salt
8 small white pickling onions, peeled
2 carrots, peeled and quartered

Preheat oven to 180° C (gas 4).

Melt butter in a large frying pan. Brown pieces of duck in fat over medium heat.

Remove to a casserole.

Add garlic to fat and cook 1 minute. Add red wine, shiitake mushrooms, parsley, bay leaf, thyme and salt. Bring to a boil, stirring constantly until sauce thickens. Place onions and carrots into casserole with duck. Top with sauce.

Cover and bake for 1¼ hours.

TOTAL GRAMS 60.4
GRAMS PER SERVING 15.1

Hal's Chicken

4 servings

1 chicken, jointed into 8 pieces
Mustard Sauce *to cover (page 184)*
1 medium onion, sliced thin
1 medium tomato, sliced thin
2 tablespoons finely chopped dill
seasoned salt to taste

Preheat oven to 180° C (gas 4).

Rinse and dry chicken. Place in a baking dish and cover with *Mustard Sauce*. Top with onion slices and then tomatoes. Sprinkle with dill and salt.

Cover and bake for 1 hour. Remove lid and bake 1 hour more.

TOTAL GRAMS 18.7
GRAMS PER SERVING 4.7

Joan's Chicken Mascarpone

4 servings

4 skinless chicken breast fillets
30 g butter
2 medium onions, sliced thin
1 clove garlic, finely chopped
½ teaspoon dried tarragon
3 tablespoons dry white wine
3 tablespoons mascarpone cheese

Preheat oven to 180° C (gas 4).

Place chicken breasts in a glass baking dish. Sauté onions, garlic, and tarragon in the butter until onions become golden. Place on top of chicken. Swirl wine in sauté pan and add mascarpone cheese. Allow cheese to melt (about 30 seconds), stir well to combine flavours and spoon over chicken and onions. Cover.

Bake for 1 hour.

TOTAL GRAMS 16.7
GRAMS PER SERVING 4.2

Tandoori Chicken

4 servings

1 2.2 kg chicken, jointed in 8 pieces
4 cloves garlic
5-cm piece root ginger, peeled
2 bay leaves
2 teaspoons chilli powder
1 teaspoon sea salt
2 teaspoons turmeric
1 teaspoon ground coriander
$\frac{1}{2}$ teaspoon ground cumin
$\frac{1}{2}$ teaspoon ground cinnamon
$\frac{1}{2}$ teaspoon ground cloves
125 ml olive oil
350 g soured cream
juice of 2 lemons

Place chicken in a covered glass baking dish large enough for pieces to lie side by side.

Place next 10 ingredients in a blender and blend to a paste.

Combine paste with soured cream and lemon juice.

Dip each piece of chicken into the mixture and coat it completely. Return chicken to baking dish.

Place in refrigerator to marinate overnight.

Bake chicken covered for 45 minutes, at 180° C (gas 4).

TOTAL GRAMS 34.2
GRAMS PER SERVING 8.6

Goat Cheesy Chicken Rolls

4 servings

4 skinless chicken breast fillets, pounded thin
60 g goat cheese, crumbled
20 g finely chopped fresh basil
1 tablespoon chopped sun-dried tomatoes in olive oil
¼ small onion, finely chopped
½ teaspoon dried oregano
½ teaspoon seasoned salt
60 ml dry white wine

Preheat oven to 180° C (gas 4).

Oil a small glass baking dish.

In a small bowl combine all ingredients except chicken and wine and blend well. Spread mixture on chicken breasts and roll them. Fasten with cocktail sticks. Arrange in baking dish so rolled breasts do not touch each other. Pour wine over chicken rolls.

Bake for 45 minutes.

TOTAL GRAMS 15.6
GRAMS PER SERVING   3.9

Oriental Chicken with Broccoli Rabe

4 servings

3 teaspoons olive oil
2 teaspoons sesame oil
2 teaspoons finely chopped root ginger
2 cloves garlic, finely chopped
4 skinless chicken breast fillets, cubed
4 large shiitake mushrooms, sliced thin
2 spring onions, finely chopped
225 g broccoli rabe, coarsely chopped
1 tablespoon Tamari soy sauce
2 tablespoons dry sherry

Heat 2 teaspoons of the olive oil and the sesame oil in a non-stick wok or frying pan. Do not allow oil to smoke. Add ginger and garlic and stir for 30 seconds. Add chicken and mushrooms and stir 3 minutes more. Remove from frying pan. Stir remaining olive oil into pan. Add spring onions and broccoli rabe. Stir-fry for 1 minute. Put back chicken and mushrooms and add soy sauce and sherry.

Remove chicken and vegetables with a slotted spoon. Place on a serving plate. Boil sauce until it reduces by half. Pour over chicken and serve immediately.

TOTAL GRAMS 32.5
GRAMS PER SERVING 8.1

Turkey Sausage Patties

8 patties

30 ml garlic oil
1 small onion, chopped fine
1 clove garlic, minced
450 g minced turkey
3 tablespoons soured cream
10 fried pork rinds, crushed
½ teaspoon finely chopped sage leaves
½ teaspoon seasoned salt
30 ml walnut oil

Heat garlic oil in a non-stick frying pan. Add onion and garlic and sauté until onions are golden.

Mix all other ingredients (except walnut oil) together in a bowl. Add onions and garlic and shape into eight balls. Flatten balls into patties. Heat walnut oil in frying pan and sauté patties until brown on both sides.

TOTAL GRAMS 7.1
GRAMS PER SERVING 0.9

Ivan's Crisp Chicken

4 servings

1 2.2 kg chicken, jointed in 8 pieces
60 ml garlic oil
60 ml white wine
1 medium-size red onion, sliced thin
seasoned salt to taste
30 g grated Jarlsberg cheese
30 g grated mature Cheddar cheese

Preheat oven to 180° C (gas 4).

Rinse and dry chicken. Brush with garlic oil. Place in baking dish and sprinkle with wine. Cover with onions. Salt to taste and bake, covered, for ½ hour.

Uncover, sprinkle with cheeses and bake uncovered until chicken, onions and cheeses are crisp, about 45 minutes.

TOTAL GRAMS 7.3
GRAMS PER SERVING 1.8

Fish and Shellfish

Sun Luck Scallops

4 servings

60 ml Tamari soy sauce
30 ml sake
450 g queen scallops
30 ml sesame oil
6 shiitake mushrooms, sliced thin
110 g soured cream

Preheat oven to 180° C (gas 4).

Mix soy sauce and sake together. Place scallops in a glass baking dish. Pour soy sauce mixture over scallops and place in refrigerator for ½ hour. Heat sesame oil in a frying pan. Sauté mushrooms for 2 minutes. Turn off heat and allow to cool in oil. Place scallops in oven and bake for 10 minutes. Spoon soured cream into a small dish. Spoon 1 tablespoon of sauce from scallops over mushrooms and artistically arrange them on top of soured cream. Enjoy eating by dipping a scallop in the mushroom and soured cream mixture.

TOTAL GRAMS 33.4
GRAMS PER SERVING 8.4

Snappy Swordfish

6 servings

1.2 kg swordfish steak
juice of 1 lemon
3 teaspoons garlic purée (available in a tube)
2 tablespoons chopped dill (or 1 tablespoon dried)
1 medium tomato, thinly sliced
225 g shiitake mushrooms, sliced
45 ml olive oil
70 g shelled sunflower seeds
225 g sugar snap peas, trimmed
60 ml dry white wine
90 g herbed goat cheese, crumbled

Preheat oven to 180° C (gas 4).

Rinse and dry swordfish. Sprinkle both sides with lemon juice and place in a covered glass baking dish.

Spread garlic purée evenly on fish. Top with dill, tomato, and mushrooms. Sprinkle olive oil and sunflower seeds evenly across the top.

Spread sugar snap peas over fish; pour wine over the peas.

Cover and place in oven for 20 minutes. Uncover, add goat cheese and cook for 10 minutes more, basting frequently.

TOTAL GRAMS 50.4
GRAMS PER SERVING 8.4

Poached Fish Fillets (Basic Recipe)

4 servings

4 fish fillets (sole, salmon, halibut, etc)
juice of 1 lemon diluted with an equal amount of water
1 small onion
½ teaspoon seasoned salt
15 g butter
3 large mushrooms, thinly sliced
60 ml water
125 ml dry white wine

Preheat oven to 180° C (gas 4).

Rinse fillets in the lemon juice and water mixture, and dry. Place in a covered glass baking dish. Melt butter in a pan over medium heat. Add mushrooms and sprinkle with seasoned salt. Cook for 2 minutes. Stir in water and wine. Bring to a boil and pour over fish. Cover, place in oven, and poach for 15 minutes. For salmon, allow 5 minutes' additional cooking time.

TOTAL GRAMS 10.4
GRAMS PER SERVING 2.6

Halibut Roll-Ups

4 servings

900 g halibut fillets
seasoned salt
3 rashers streaky bacon, diced
125 g shiitake mushrooms, sliced
30 g celery, diced
20 g onion, diced
1 clove garlic, finely chopped
1 tablespoon chopped parsley
45 g unsalted butter, melted
125 ml dry white wine
20 g Parmesan cheese, grated
paprika to taste

Preheat oven to 180° C (gas 4).

Sprinkle fillets with salt. Allow to stand for about 10 minutes. Place in a glass baking dish.

In frying pan, sauté bacon, mushrooms, celery and onion until vegetables are soft and bacon is crisp. Add garlic and cook 2 minutes more. Add parsley and blend well.

Spread mixture over fillets, roll up, and fasten with cocktail sticks. Place one third of melted butter in bottom of baking dish. Add fish. Pour remaining butter over fish, and add wine.

Sprinkle with Parmesan cheese and paprika.

Bake for ½ hour.

TOTAL GRAMS 11.6
GRAMS PER SERVING 2.9

Sole with Soured Cream

6 servings

1.4 kg sole fillets (or plaice)
lemon juice
salt and pepper
1 teaspoon dried tarragon
450 g soured cream
1 tablespoon chopped chives and parsley

Preheat oven to 180° C (gas 4).

Oil a baking dish just large enough to hold fish fillets. Rub fillets with lemon juice, salt and pepper, and place in dish.

Sprinkle with tarragon. Cover with soured cream and bake for 20 minutes, or until fish flakes easily.

Remove from oven and sprinkle with chives and parsley. Serve immediately.

TOTAL GRAMS 22.5
GRAMS PER SERVING 3.8

Stuffed Sole

6 servings

900 g lemon sole fillets, skinned
salt to taste
3 rashers streaky bacon, diced
125 g shiitake mushrooms, sliced
30 g diced celery
20 g diced onion
1 clove garlic, finely chopped
1 tablespoon chopped parsley
45 g butter, melted
125 ml dry white wine
20 g Parmesan cheese, grated
paprika

Preheat oven to 180° C (gas 4).

Sprinkle fillets with salt. Allow to stand for about 10 minutes.

Sauté bacon, mushrooms, celery and onion in a non-stick frying pan until vegetables are soft and bacon crisp. Add garlic. Cook for 2 minutes more. Add parsley and blend well.

Spread mixture over fillets, roll them up, and fasten with cocktail sticks. Place one third of melted butter in bottom of baking dish. Add fish.

Pour remaining butter over fish, and add wine.

Sprinkle with Parmesan cheese and paprika.

Bake for ½ hour.

TOTAL GRAMS 11.7
GRAMS PER SERVING 2.0

Fennel Red Mullet

4 servings

4 fillets of red mullet or snapper, about 675 g
60 g butter, softened
1 teaspoon fennel seeds
½ teaspoon lemon juice
¼ teaspoon dried tarragon
1 clove garlic, finely chopped
seasoned salt to taste
60 ml olive oil
1 teaspoon grated lemon zest
½ bay leaf

Rinse and dry fish. Combine butter, fennel seeds, lemon juice, tarragon, garlic and salt. Spread butter mixture on fish fillets, roll them up, and fasten with cocktail sticks.

Combine oil, lemon zest, and bay leaf in baking dish. Add fish and marinate in refrigerator for 1 hour. Turn once. Drain fish and reserve marinade.

Preheat oven to 180° C (gas 4).

Bake for 45 minutes. Serve with warmed marinade on side.

TOTAL GRAMS 1.5
GRAMS PER SERVING 0.4

Trout in Tomato Sauce

4 servings

4 trout fillets, about 675 g
75 ml prepared tomato sauce or passata
120 ml cider vinegar
45 ml olive oil
10 g finely chopped onion
4 drops Tabasco sauce (optional)
1 teaspoon sugar substitute (optional)

Cut fish into 1-cm pieces. Arrange attractively in shallow serving dish.

Combine remaining ingredients. Mix well. Pour over fish and cover. Place in refrigerator for 24 hours.

Preheat oven to 180° C (gas 4).

Bake, uncovered for 45 minutes.

TOTAL GRAMS 13.4
GRAMS PER SERVING 3.4

Fresh Spring Salmon Mousse

10 servings

15 g (2 tablespoons) gelatine
375 ml cold water
150 g soured cream
220 g mayonnaise
675 g fresh salmon, cooked, skinned, and boned
½ teaspoon onion powder
1 tablespoon capers, drained
2 teaspoons chopped dill
120 g cucumber, peeled, de-seeded and chopped
1 teaspoon salt

Soften gelatine in cold water. Heat until completely dissolved. Cool.

Mix soured cream and mayonnaise together. Add gelatine and chill until slightly thickened.

Flake salmon and add onion powder, capers, dill, cucumber and salt. Mix well with soured cream and mayonnaise.

Pour into 1.25-litre capacity mould. Refrigerate until firm.

Unmould and serve.

TOTAL GRAMS 17.4
GRAMS PER SERVING 1.7

Tuna Loaf

4 servings

500 g canned tuna, drained, or 450 g fresh tuna, poached, skinned and boned
10 g finely chopped onion
2 teaspoons capers
220 g mayonnaise
125 ml water
125 ml whipping cream
½ teaspoon salt
¼ teaspoon paprika
½ teaspoon curry, or to taste

Preheat oven to 180° C (gas 4).

Drain fish. In a small bowl flake fish. Add onion and capers to fish.

Combine mayonnaise, water, cream, salt and paprika. Stir until smooth.

Add half the sauce to fish and mix. Place mixture in buttered loaf tin or baking dish. Bake for 30 minutes.

Add curry to remaining sauce. To serve, slice fish loaf and spoon sauce over slices.

TOTAL GRAMS 8.4
GRAMS PER SERVING 2.1

Oriental Prawns

2 servings

30 g butter
25 g onion, chopped
3 slices boiled ham, cut into strips
1 clove garlic, finely chopped
50 g bean sprouts
¼ head cabbage, shredded
450 g raw prawns, shelled and deveined
4 servings Fish Stock *(page 71)*
paprika

Preheat oven to 180° C (gas 4).

Melt butter in saucepan, add onion, and sauté until soft. Add ham and garlic, and sauté for 3 minutes. Add bean sprouts, and sauté for about 3 or 4 minutes until lightly browned.

Place prawns in small casserole. Add uncooked cabbage to bean sprout mixture. Spread over prawns.

Pour *Fish Stock* over all. Sprinkle with paprika. Cover dish with lid or aluminium foil and bake for 30 minutes.

TOTAL GRAMS 21.6
GRAMS PER SERVING 5.4

Prawns Parmesan

4 servings

30 ml olive oil
80 g onion, finely chopped
2 cloves garlic, finely chopped
900 g raw prawns, shelled and deveined
225 g prepared tomato sauce or passata
1 teaspoon dried basil
¼ teaspoon dried oregano
2 teaspoons salt
pepper to taste
225 g shredded mozzarella cheese
20 g Parmesan cheese, grated

Preheat grill.

Heat 1 tablespoon oil in frying pan. Sauté onion until golden, add garlic, and sauté 1 minute.

Add prawns and sauté for 3 minutes, remove from pan and place in a baking dish.

In frying pan, heat remainder of oil, add passata, oregano and basil. Simmer for 15 minutes. Salt and pepper to taste.

Pour over prawns and add shredded mozzarella cheese on top. Top with Parmesan and grill until bubbly.

TOTAL GRAMS 32.6
GRAMS PER SERVING 8.1

Prawns and Scallops Marc

2 servings

450 g medium prawns, shelled and deveined
generous dash seasoned salt
generous dash garlic powder
1 egg, beaten
20 g Parmesan cheese, grated
450 g scallops
125 ml whipping cream
30 g unsalted butter
3 rashers diced bacon, cooked
60 ml dry white wine
tarragon sprigs

Sprinkle prawns with salt and garlic powder. Dip prawns in egg and then coat with Parmesan cheese.

Sprinkle scallops with additional salt and garlic powder, dip into cream, and then coat with Parmesan cheese. Reserve remaining cream.

Melt butter in pan. Add bacon, scallops and prawns. Brown on both sides; add wine and simmer for 10 minutes. Add reserved cream and simmer gently for 10 minutes longer. Garnish with tarragon.

Total Grams 13.6
Grams per Serving   6.8

Tarragon Lobster Tails

2 servings

4 lobster tails, thawed if frozen
60 g butter
1 tablespoon chopped fresh ginger (or 1 teaspoon ground)
1 teaspoon dried tarragon
½ teaspoon dry mustard
seasoned salt

Preheat grill.

Remove soft part of lobster tail/carapace with scissors. Hit hard shell slightly with mallet or cleaver to make it lie flat. Melt butter. Add ginger, tarragon, mustard and salt. Spoon generously over tails and allow to stand 20 minutes.

Grill about 10 cm from heat for 10–15 minutes with meaty side up. Baste often.

TOTAL GRAMS 2.8
GRAMS PER SERVING 1.4

Crab and Almond Pie

8 servings

40 g chopped toasted almonds (see Toasted Nuts *recipe, page 68)*
2 eggs plus 2 egg yolks
2 teaspoons Dijon mustard
2 teaspoons seasoned salt
2 tablespoons chopped chives
225 g grated fontina cheese
115 g frozen or canned, drained crab meat
375 ml whipping cream

Preheat oven to 150° C (gas 2).

Place toasted almonds on the bottom of 23-cm shallow pie dish or ceramic quiche mould.

Put eggs and yolks in bowl and beat well. Add mustard, salt, chives, cheese and crab meat.

Scald cream by bringing it right to the boiling point (do not boil).
Add cream to mixture and pour into pie dish.
Bake for 1 hour.

TOTAL GRAMS 40.7
GRAMS PER SERVING 5.1

Curried Crab

4 servings

120 g onion, chopped
60 ml olive oil
2 tablespoons curry powder
450 g crab meat, flaked and picked over
2 tablespoons chopped parsley
¼ teaspoon crushed red pepper flakes
30 ml lemon juice
½ teaspoon seasoned salt
½ teaspoon black pepper
¼ teaspoon dried oregano
60 g grated Parmesan cheese
30 g butter
1 lemon, cut into wedges

Preheat grill.

Sauté onion in oil until soft. Add curry powder and cook, stirring constantly, for 1 minute.

Stir in crab meat, parsley and red pepper, and sauté for 2 minutes. Add lemon juice, salt, pepper and oregano. Sauté for 1 minute more.

Divide crab mixture among 4 buttered scallop shells or small ramekins, sprinkle each serving with Parmesan cheese, and dot tops with butter. Place under grill for 2–3 minutes, or until cheese is golden. Serve with lemon wedges.

TOTAL GRAMS 26.6
GRAMS PER SERVING 6.7

Houston's Ceviche

4 servings

450 g whitefish (or trout), cut into bite-sized pieces
450 g medium prawns, shelled and deveined
450 g queen scallops
juice of 6 limes
juice of 4 lemons
3 tablespoons finely chopped garlic
6 slices peeled ginger root
1 medium onion, sliced thin
1 teaspoon chopped coriander

Rinse and dry fish and shellfish. Mix all remaining ingredients together. Place in a glass baking dish just large enough to hold fish, prawns and scallops. Mix fish, shellfish and citrus mixture and refrigerate for 2 days until fish and shellfish "cook." The fish and shellfish will be opaque and appear to have been cooked.

Serve cold.

TOTAL GRAMS 49.6
GRAMS PER SERVING 12.4

Pasta

Manicotti

12 crepes

1 recipe Pasta Sauce *(pages 182–3)*
1 recipe Pasta *(page 159)*
Stuffing for Pasta:
450 g ricotta cheese
180 g mozzarella cheese
2 teaspoons chopped parsley
5 tablespoons grated Parmesan cheese
2 eggs

Preheat oven to 150° C (gas 2).

Prepare 1.75 litres *Pasta Sauce* and 12 *Pasta Crepes*; set aside.

In a bowl mix ricotta cheese, mozzarella cheese, parsley, 2 tablespoons of the Parmesan cheese, and eggs.

Cover the bottom of large baking dish with thin layer of *Pasta Sauce.*

Place about 3 full tablespoons of ricotta mixture in centre of a crepe. Roll crepe around stuffing. Place crepe in baking dish, seam side down. Repeat with each crepe, placing them side by side in baking pan. Pour remaining sauce over crepes.

Sprinkle remaining 3 tablespoons Parmesan cheese on top. Bake for 20 minutes.

TOTAL GRAMS 97.0
GRAMS PER MANICOTTI 7.6

Gnocchi

8 servings

450 g ricotta cheese, pressed of liquid
225 g full fat soft (cream) cheese or Boursin cheese
3 eggs, beaten
15 g soy flour
dash of salt, cayenne pepper and nutmeg
225 g unsalted butter, melted
50 g Parmesan cheese, grated

Push ricotta cheese and soft cheese through a fine strainer. (The easiest and fastest way is with your hands.)

Beat eggs into mixture with electric or rotary beater. Blend in soy flour and seasonings. Refrigerate for about 1 hour. Bring large pot of water to rolling boil. Lower heat to simmer. Drop cheese mixture into water by teaspoonfuls. (They will drop and then rise to the top.)

Allow gnocchi to poach (simmer on top of water) for about 20 minutes. Remove gnocchi carefully with a slotted spoon and allow to drain on kitchen paper.

Put half the butter in large baking dish. Place drained gnocchi in dish. Cover with remaining melted butter and grated Parmesan cheese.

Gnocchi may be served immediately, kept warm in a low oven or refrigerated and reheated.

The substitution of Boursin for cream cheese will give you a much spicier gnocchi. Adding 70 g of frozen spinach that has been thawed and squeezed dry makes a delicious Spinach Gnocchi.

TOTAL GRAMS 27.2
GRAMS PER SERVING 3.4

Enchiladas

6 servings

1 recipe Pasta *(page 159)*
675 g minced pork
3 cloves garlic, finely chopped
3 teaspoons chilli powder
45 ml cider vinegar
15 ml oil
30 g chopped onion
250 ml prepared tomato sauce or passata
250 ml water
½ teaspoon ground cumin
1 teaspoon chilli powder
6 drops Tabasco sauce, or to taste
1 teaspoon salt, or to taste
170 g grated Cheddar cheese

Prepare *Pasta* recipe. Place *Pasta* on greaseproof paper, and set aside.
Preheat oven to 180° C (gas 4).

In bowl combine minced pork, garlic, 2 teaspoons of the chilli powder and vinegar.

Heat oil in frying pan, and sauté onion over medium heat for 3 or 4 minutes until soft.

Add pork mixture to onion, and brown. Cook thoroughly. Pour off all fat. Set aside.

Sauce:

In saucepan combine tomato sauce, water, cumin, chilli powder, Tabasco sauce and salt. Simmer for ½ hour.

Pour 125 ml sauce in a 32 cm × 23 cm baking dish. Fill crepes with 2 tablespoons pork mixture and 1 tablespoon cheese. Fold over and place crepes seam side down in baking dish. Repeat until you use all crepes. Pour remaining sauce over all. Bake for 15 minutes. Cover with remaining cheese. Bake for 5 minutes more or until cheese is hot and bubbly.

TOTAL GRAMS 44.4
GRAMS PER SERVING 7.4

Pasta

12 crepes

45 g soy flour
125 ml water
3 eggs
15 ml oil

Put all ingredients in blender. Blend until smooth. Use a crepe pan or a 13- or 15-cm frying pan. Cover bottom of pan lightly with small amount of oil. When pan is hot enough to sizzle a drop of water, pour about 3 tablespoons of crepe mixture into pan. Tilt pan to distribute mixture evenly. Crepes should be thin. Lightly brown on both sides (about 1 minute on each side). Stack between greaseproof paper until all crepes are finished.

The crepes are very delicate, so handle carefully. If you have trouble the first time, try again. Oil pan again if necessary.

They can be made a day ahead and stored in refrigerator separated by sheets of greaseproof paper.

TOTAL GRAMS 10.8
GRAMS PER SERVING 0.9

Cannelloni

4 servings

3 chicken livers
1 chicken breast fillet
60 g butter
5 thin slices prosciutto ham
¼ teaspoon dried marjoram
75 g grated Parmesan cheese
1 recipe Cream Sauce *(page 180)*
1 recipe Pasta *(page 159)*

Preheat oven to 120° C (gas ¾).

Sauté chicken livers and chicken breast in butter over medium heat until brown on both sides. Grind livers, chicken breast and prosciutto in food grinder with medium blade. Mix in marjoram and 50 g of the grated Parmesan cheese. Add 150 ml of the *Cream Sauce*. Place 2 tablespoons chicken mixture in centre of each crepe. Roll up crepes.

Butter baking dish and place crepes seam side down. Cover with remaining sauce and Parmesan cheese. Bake for 15 minutes.

TOTAL GRAMS 13.0
GRAMS PER SERVING 3.3

Bread

4 Grain and Seed Bread

12 slices

1 tablespoon plain flour
1 tablespoon wholewheat flour
1 tablespoon maize flour
1 tablespoon sesame seeds
½ teaspoon baking powder
2 eggs, separated
2 teaspoons sugar substitute
⅛ teaspoon seasoned salt
2 tablespoons full fat ricotta cheese
30 g butter
⅛ teaspoon cream of tartar
1 tablespoon pumpkin seeds

Preheat oven to 180° C (gas 4).

Mix flours, sesame seeds and baking powder together. Beat in egg yolks. Sprinkle with sugar substitute and seasoned salt. Mix cheese with butter. Add dry ingredients to cheese mixture and blend well.

Whisk egg whites with cream of tartar until stiff. Fold into cheese mixture.

Spoon into a small, oiled loaf tin. Sprinkle with pumpkin seeds and bake for 50 minutes. Cool on a wire rack.

TOTAL GRAMS 24.6
GRAMS PER SERVING 2.1

Rye Bread

12 slices

2 tablespoons plain flour
1 tablespoon wholewheat flour
1 tablespoon rye flour
1 tablespoon caraway seeds
½ teaspoon baking powder
2 teaspoons sugar substitute
2 eggs, separated
⅛ teaspoon seasoned salt
2 tablespoons ricotta cheese
30 g butter, melted
⅛ teaspoon cream of tartar

Preheat oven to 180° C (gas 4).

Mix flours and caraway seeds together. Beat in egg yolks and sprinkle with seasoned salt and sugar substitute. Mix cheese with butter, add dry ingredients, and blend well. Whisk egg whites with cream of tartar until stiff. Fold into cheese mixture. Spoon into a small oiled loaf tin and bake for 50 minutes. Remove from oven and cool on rack.

TOTAL GRAMS 23.7
GRAMS PER SERVING 2.0

Courgette Bread

12 slices

2 tablespoons plain flour
1 tablespoon wholewheat flour
160 g courgettes, grated and pressed to remove liquid
½ teaspoon baking powder
¼ teaspoon seasoned salt
2 teaspoons sugar substitute
2 eggs, separated
2 tablespoons ricotta cheese
2 tablespoons grated Parmesan cheese
⅛ teaspoon cream of tartar
10 walnuts

Preheat oven to 180° C (gas 4).

Mix flours, salt, sugar substitute, baking powder and courgette. Beat in one egg yolk at a time. Mix in ricotta and Parmesan cheeses. Beat egg whites with cream of tartar until stiff. Fold into cheese mixture. Spoon into small loaf tin and place walnut halves on top.

Bake for 50 minutes. Remove from oven and cool on a rack.

TOTAL GRAMS 34.7
GRAMS PER SERVING 2.9

Vegetables

Aubergine Parmigiana

8 servings

1 large aubergine, cut into 1-cm slices
60 ml olive oil
1 large onion, chopped
2 cloves garlic, finely chopped
450 g minced steak
250 ml prepared tomato sauce, or passata
250 ml water
1 teaspoon oregano
50 g Parmesan cheese, grated
450 g mozzarella cheese, sliced

Preheat oven to 180° C (gas 4).

Soak aubergine in salted water for 1 hour. Dry with kitchen paper.

Heat half the olive oil in a frying pan and lightly brown chopped onion. Add garlic and sauté one more minute. Add minced steak, stir and cook. When meat turns brown, add tomato sauce and water. Simmer for 15 minutes. Place remaining olive oil in a separate large frying pan over medium heat and sauté a few aubergine slices at a time until golden brown; add a little more oil if needed.

Oil a baking dish and arrange half of the aubergine slices on the bottom. Cover with half of the tomato-meat mixture. Sprinkle with half of the Parmesan cheese and half of the mozzarella. Repeat these layers.

Bake for 25 to 30 minutes until golden brown.

TOTAL GRAMS 62.6
GRAMS PER SERVING 7.8

Broccoli with Cheese Sauce

6 servings

450 g broccoli
1 recipe Cheese Sauce *(page 186)*

Prepare broccoli by removing hard stem and reserving florets. Place in a steamer and steam for 10 to 15 minutes, depending on how soft you like your vegetables. Serve with *Cheese Sauce* (3 tablespoons per serving).

TOTAL GRAMS 35.7
GRAMS PER SERVING 5.9

Baked Spinach

4 servings

140 g cooked spinach (from 340 g fresh)
45 ml olive oil
45 g butter
30 g onion, finely chopped
1 clove garlic, finely chopped
2 slices prosciutto, diced
5 eggs
45 ml whipping cream
pinch of black pepper
20 g grated Parmesan cheese

Preheat oven to 180° C (gas 4).

Heat olive oil and butter in frying pan.

Add onion, garlic and prosciutto to frying pan. Cook slowly until onion is light brown. Add onion mixture to spinach and place in a baking dish.

Beat eggs with cream and add pepper. Pour over spinach. Sprinkle with Parmesan cheese.

Bake for 30 minutes, or until set.

TOTAL GRAMS 13.9
GRAMS PER SERVING 3.5

Stuffed Zippy Courgettes

4 servings

2 medium-size courgettes
90 g ricotta cheese
1 teaspoon chopped parsley
1 onion, chopped
1 egg white, whisked stiff
250 ml prepared tomato sauce or passata

Preheat oven to 150° C (gas 2).

Cut courgettes into halves lengthways and scoop out pulp, leaving a 1-cm shell.

Combine ricotta, parsley and onion. Mix well. Fold in egg white.

Stuff mixture into halved courgettes. Place in baking dish and pour tomato sauce over top.

Bake for 10 minutes. Lower heat to 120° C (gas ³/₄). and cook for 30 more minutes. Baste often.

TOTAL GRAMS 42.7
GRAMS PER SERVING 10.7

Stuffed Courgettes with Prosciutto

6 servings

6 medium-size courgettes
45 g mayonnaise
15 g grated Parmesan cheese
40 g mushrooms, sliced
4 slices lean prosciutto, diced
1 egg yolk
1 teaspoon salt
¹/₂ teaspoon pepper
¹/₂ teaspoon dried oregano
45 ml olive oil

Preheat oven to 190° C (gas 5).

Cut courgettes into halves lengthways. Scoop out pulp and reserve.

Mix together pulp from courgettes, mayonnaise, Parmesan cheese, mushrooms, prosciutto, egg yolk, salt, pepper and oregano.

Place courgette halves in greased baking dish and fill each courgette half with mixture. Sprinkle with olive oil. Bake for 30 minutes.

TOTAL GRAMS 50.6
GRAMS PER SERVING 8.4

Green Beans Amandine

4 servings

450 g fresh or frozen stringless green beans
225 g shiitake mushrooms, sliced
60 g butter
½ teaspoon seasoned salt
30 g sliced almonds

Top and tail beans, if needed. Simmer in small amount of water for 10 minutes. In a frying pan, sauté mushrooms in butter until brown. Add salt and almonds.

Add beans to pan. Toss well. Simmer for 4 minutes. Correct seasoning to taste.

TOTAL GRAMS 43.2
GRAMS PER SERVING 10.8

Cauliflower Cheese Dumplings

12 dumplings

½ head cauliflower (about 450 g)
2 eggs, beaten
50 g grated Parmesan cheese
1 teaspoon chopped parsley
1 teaspoon grated nutmeg
30 g soy flour
1 tablespoon salt, for cooking
60 g butter

Boil cauliflower until soft, about 25 minutes. Mash with fork or potato masher. (Should be about 200 g mashed.)

Add eggs, Parmesan cheese, parsley, nutmeg and soy flour. Shape into walnut-size balls.

Bring large pot of water to rolling boil. Add salt. Drop cauliflower balls into water. When they rise, remove with slotted spoon.

Heat butter in frying pan. Fry balls until brown on all sides. Drain on kitchen paper.

TOTAL GRAMS 18.1
GRAMS PER SERVING 1.5

Chinese Mangetout

6 servings

30 ml vegetable oil
1 onion, chopped fine
1 clove garlic, chopped fine
½ teaspoon seasoned salt
35 g sliced water chestnuts
225 g mangetouts
15 ml Tamari soy sauce
60 ml Chicken Stock *(page 69)*

Heat oil in heavy frying pan. Add onion, garlic, salt and water chestnuts. Sauté until onion is golden. Add mangetouts, soy sauce and *Chicken Stock*. Cover and cook for 5 minutes. Uncover and cook for 5 more minutes.

TOTAL GRAMS 28.4
GRAMS PER SERVING 4.7

Aubergine "Little Shoes"

8 servings

4 medium aubergines
30 g butter
40 g onion, chopped
1 clove garlic, finely chopped
450 g minced beef or lamb
250 ml prepared tomato sauce or passata
1 teaspoon ground cumin
1 teaspoon chopped parsley
1 teaspoon seasoned salt
pepper to taste
1 egg
15 ml water
15 ml lemon juice
25g grated Parmesan cheese

Preheat oven to 180° C (gas 4).

Wash aubergines. Do not peel. Parboil whole aubergines in salted boiling water for 5 minutes. Remove. Cut in half lengthways. Spoon out centre pulp carefully and chop, leaving about 5-mm shell.

Melt butter in saucepan. Add onion and garlic. Sauté for 3 minutes. Add meat and aubergine pulp. Stir. Brown lightly. Add tomato sauce, cumin, parsley, salt and pepper. Cook over low heat until all liquid is absorbed.

Place aubergine shells in lightly oiled roasting tin or large casserole dish. Stuff with meat mixture. Beat egg, water and lemon juice together. Pour over aubergines. Sprinkle with Parmesan cheese. Bake for 20 minutes until lightly browned.

TOTAL GRAMS 57.2
GRAMS PER SERVING 7.2

Cheese-Stuffed Aubergine

8 servings

4 medium-size aubergines
2 medium-size onions, chopped
45 g butter
330 g feta cheese, crumbled
50 g grated Parmesan cheese
60 g ricotta cheese
1 egg
2 tablespoons chopped parsley
seasoned salt

Preheat oven to 180° C (gas 4).

Slice aubergines in half. Scoop out pulp, chop it, and set aside. Reserve shells. Sauté onions in butter until golden. Add aubergine pulp and continue to sauté for about 5 more minutes. Transfer mixture to bowl and let cool. Add cheeses to mixture; beat in egg and parsley. Stuff mixture in aubergine shells. Sprinkle with salt. Bake for 40 minutes.

TOTAL GRAMS 62.3
GRAMS PER SERVING 7.8

The Most Delicious Cucumbers

4 servings

4 cucumbers, peeled and de-seeded
1½ teaspoons seasoned salt
1½ teaspoons tarragon vinegar
60 g butter, melted
1 tablespoon chopped dill
1 tablespoon chopped chives
1 tablespoon chopped onion
60 ml whipping cream
2 tablespoons chopped parsley
grated Parmesan cheese

Preheat oven to 190° C (gas 5).

Slice cucumbers to bite-size pieces. Add salt and vinegar. Allow to stand at room temperature for at least 2 hours. Drain and dry thoroughly with kitchen paper.

Put cucumbers in casserole with butter, dill, chives and onion. Bake for 25 minutes.

Remove from oven; add whipping cream. Stir over medium heat on top of stove for about 5 minutes (do not allow to boil). Cream will thicken. Sprinkle with parsley and small amount of Parmesan cheese. Serve hot.

TOTAL GRAMS 23.2
GRAMS PER SERVING 5.8

Crazy Cabbage

8 servings

1 cabbage, trimmed
1 onion, chopped
120 g bacon, diced
2 garlic cloves, finely chopped
30 ml olive oil
4 tablespoons chopped parsley
1 egg
1 tablespoon grated Parmesan cheese
250 ml Chicken Stock *(page 69)*
seasoned salt

Preheat oven to 190° C (gas 5).

Boil cabbage in salted water for 15 minutes. Remove and run under cold water. Core cabbage, leaving outer leaves intact. Chop core and inner leaves. Sauté cabbage, onion, bacon and garlic together in olive oil.

Mix parsley with egg and Parmesan cheese. Beat well.

Mix egg mixture into sautéed cabbage.

Oil a deep casserole. Place large outer cabbage leaves in casserole. Fill middle with sautéed mixture. Pour *Chicken Stock* over mixture. Add seasoned salt to taste. Cover and bake for 1 hour. Remove cover and bake for 30 more minutes. Serve.

TOTAL GRAMS 37.4
GRAMS PER SERVING 4.7

Ratatouille

12 90-g servings

65 ml olive oil
3 medium-size courgettes, unpeeled, quartered, cut into 2.5-cm lengths
½ medium-size aubergine, unpeeled, cut into 4-cm cubes
salt and pepper to taste
2 medium-size onions, chopped
5 cloves garlic, finely chopped
2 green peppers, de-seeded and chopped
250 ml prepared tomato sauce or passata
½ teaspoon dried thyme
1 teaspoon dried basil
4 tablespoons finely chopped parsley
lemon wedges

Preheat oven to 180° C (gas 4).

Heat 25 ml of the olive oil in large frying pan, add courgettes, aubergine, salt and pepper. Cook, stirring occasionally, for about 10 minutes.

Heat remaining olive oil in another frying pan. Add onions, garlic and peppers, and cook until lightly browned. Add tomato sauce and simmer, stirring occasionally, for about 10 minutes.

Add courgette and aubergine mixture, then thyme, basil and parsley. Pour in casserole, cover, and bake for about 20 minutes, or until vegetables are tender.

Can be served warm, or cold with lemon wedges.

TOTAL GRAMS 73.7
GRAMS PER SERVING 6.1

Basic Fried Green Tomatoes

Not always available, I treat green tomatoes like jewels when I have them. The following recipes are easy to prepare and enjoy.

1 green tomato, washed and sliced
15 ml garlic oil
15 g unsalted butter

Heat garlic oil and butter together in small non-stick frying pan. Place tomato slices in frying pan and fry over medium heat on both sides until brown.

TOTAL GRAMS 6.3

Variation 1: Sprinkle with sugar substitute while cooking.
Variation 2: Sprinkle with seasoned salt while cooking.
Variation 3: Dip tomatoes in egg and then in grated Parmesan cheese before frying.

TOTAL GRAMS 7.3

Variation 4: Spoon ½ teaspoon of white wine on each slice as it cooks.

TOTAL GRAMS 6.5

Variation 5: When finished frying, place a slice of Gruyère cheese and crumbled bacon on top of each slice and grill until cheese begins to bubble.

TOTAL GRAMS 6.4

Variation 6: Top with warm goat cheese and serve on lettuce, garnished with ½ avocado for a delicious lunch salad.

TOTAL GRAMS 13.6

Porcini Mushrooms

4 servings

4 large porcini mushrooms
30 g butter
30 ml garlic oil
30 ml white wine
4 tablespoons mascarpone cheese
2 tablespoons Tamari soy sauce

Rinse and dry mushrooms and cut off stems, leaving caps intact. (You can keep stems for another use.)

Heat butter and garlic oil in a large frying pan. Add mushrooms and cook for 3 minutes over medium heat. Turn once. Add wine to the pan. Turn mushrooms again. Place 1 tablespoon of mascarpone cheese in centre of each mushroom. Sprinkle with soy sauce. Cook 1 minute longer and serve hot.

TOTAL GRAMS 12.6
GRAMS PER SERVING 3.2

Cauliflower Bake

6 servings

30 g butter
½ onion, finely chopped
4 cloves garlic, finely chopped
225 g cauliflower, chopped
2 eggs, beaten
100 g Parmesan cheese, grated
5 rashers streaky bacon, cooked crisp and crumbled

Preheat oven to 180° C (gas 4).

Heat butter in a frying pan. Add onions and garlic and cook until onions turn golden. Add cauliflower and continue to cook 1 minute more. Remove to a bowl. Add eggs, Parmesan cheese and crumbled bacon.

Spoon into a buttered baking dish. Bake for 1 hour, or until brown.

TOTAL GRAMS 21.5
GRAMS PER SERVING 3.6

Crispy White Radish

2 servings

1 medium daikon (white radish)
garlic oil
seasoned salt

Using the large holes on a four-sided grater, shred radish. Fill a 23-cm frying pan ¼ full with garlic oil. Heat oil until very hot. Fry radish until golden brown. Remove from oil with slotted spoon and drain on kitchen or brown paper. Sprinkle with seasoned salt.

Better than French fries!

TOTAL GRAMS 3.6
GRAMS PER SERVING 1.8

Cheesy Brussels Sprouts

4 servings

20 Brussels sprouts, washed and trimmed
garlic oil
2 tablespoons grated Parmesan cheese

Slice Brussels sprouts in half. Heat enough garlic oil to ¼ fill a frying pan. Fry Brussels sprouts until golden on both sides.

Remove with a slotted spoon and allow to drain on kitchen or brown paper. Place in a bowl and toss with Parmesan cheese.

TOTAL GRAMS 34.4
GRAMS PER SERVING 8.6

Swede Home Fries

6 servings

½ large swede, peeled and quartered
30 g unsalted butter
2 medium-size onions, sliced thin
5 shiitake mushrooms, sliced thin

Boil swede in water until fork-soft. Drain and return to pan. Heat 2 minutes more to dry. Slice to size of fifty pence coins.

Melt butter in a non-stick frying pan. Add onions and sauté until transparent. Add mushrooms and continue sautéing until soft. Add swedes and sauté until brown and crisp.

TOTAL GRAMS 51.1
GRAMS PER SERVING 8.5

Irene's Turnips

4 servings

4 medium-size turnips, trimmed
seasoned salt to taste
30 g unsalted butter
3 rashers streaky bacon

Boil turnips in salted water until fork-soft. Drain well and, using a potato masher, mash turnips with butter until smooth. Cook bacon in a non-stick frying pan. Remove bacon and leave fat in pan. Spoon turnips into pan and sauté in bacon fat until turnips absorb fat. Remove to a bowl, crumble bacon on top and serve.

TOTAL GRAMS 38.6
GRAMS PER SERVING 9.7

Chic Asparagus

4 servings

450 g asparagus
45 ml extra-virgin olive oil
30 ml white wine
60 g goat cheese
2 sun-dried tomatoes in olive oil, finely chopped

Preheat oven to 180° C (gas 4).

Wash and trim asparagus, and place in a glass baking dish. Mix olive oil and wine together and sprinkle over asparagus. Dot with goat cheese and sun-dried tomatoes. Cover and bake for 15 minutes or until vegetables are tender.

TOTAL GRAMS 21.4
GRAMS PER SERVING 5.4

Green Bean Chokes

4 servings

450 g green beans
1 180-g jar marinated artichoke hearts, undrained
60 g Parmesan cheese shavings

Preheat oven to 180° C (gas 4).

Wash green beans and cut off ends. Place in a glass baking dish. Top with marinade from artichokes. Quarter artichoke hearts and spread over beans. Add Parmesan shavings. Cover and bake for 15 minutes, or until vegetables are tender.

TOTAL GRAMS 43.2
GRAMS PER SERVING 10.8

Sauces

Cream Sauce

360 ml

120 g unsalted butter
3 egg yolks
60 ml water
60 ml whipping cream
dash of nutmeg

Place butter in top of double boiler over hot (not boiling) water. Add egg yolks one at a time. Beat constantly with rotary or hand electric beater. Add water and cream. Continue to beat until sauce thickens, about 7 to 10 minutes. Add nutmeg as a garnish.

TOTAL GRAMS 4.1
GRAMS PER 15 ML/1 TABLESPOON 0.2

Frozen Horseradish Cream

285 ml

250 ml whipping cream
2 tablespoons grated horseradish
1 teaspoon seasoned salt
2 teaspoons Dijon mustard

Whip cream until stiff.

Mix together horseradish, salt and mustard. Carefully fold mixture into whipped cream. Freeze until firm.

TOTAL GRAMS 10.5
GRAMS PER 15 ML/1 TABLESPOON 0.6

Hollandaise Sauce

360 ml

30 ml tarragon vinegar
½ teaspoon seasoned salt
15 ml cold water
4 egg yolks
225 g butter, at room temperature
1 teaspoon lemon juice
15 ml whipping cream

Combine vinegar and salt in saucepan and cook rapidly to reduce by half. Remove from heat and add water. Place yolks in saucepan and beat with wire whisk until creamy. Place pan over double boiler and add butter a little at a time, beating with whisk as butter is melting. When sauce is thick, add lemon juice and cream. Beat again. Keep warm until ready to serve.

TOTAL GRAMS 3.0
GRAMS PER 15 ML/1 TABLESPOON 0.1

Tartare Sauce

225 ml

160 g mayonnaise
15 ml tarragon vinegar
1 teaspoon finely chopped onion
1 teaspoon capers, drained
1 teaspoon finely chopped cornichons
1 teaspoon finely chopped olives
1 teaspoon finely chopped parsley

Combine all ingredients. Mix well.
Store in covered jar in refrigerator. Will keep for several weeks.

TOTAL GRAMS 4.6
GRAMS PER 15 ML/1 TABLESPOON 0.3

Cocktail Sauce

240 ml

250 ml prepared tomato sauce
1 tablespoon horseradish
1 teaspoon Worcestershire sauce
1 teaspoon lemon juice

Mix all ingredients. Chill thoroughly.

TOTAL GRAMS 19.2
GRAMS PER 15 ML/1 TABLESPOON 1.2

Pasta Sauce

24 125-ml servings

2 pork chops
75 ml olive oil
1.5 litres passata
750 ml water
3 large cloves garlic, finely chopped
1 teaspoon salt
450 g mild or hot Italian sausages
450 g minced beef
1 teaspoon dried oregano
1 teaspoon dried thyme
2–4 teaspoons sugar substitute, to taste

Place pork chops and 30 ml of the olive oil in a large heavy pot. Brown chops well. Add passata, water, garlic and salt.

Bring to slow boil. Allow to simmer.

Meanwhile, place sausages in heavy frying pan without any oil. Prick sausages with fork. Cook until well browned on all sides. Slice into 1-cm pieces. Drain well and discard drippings. Add sausage pieces to pork chop mixture.

Brown minced beef in frying pan with remaining olive oil. As mince is browning, slowly break up into small pieces. When it is lightly browned, add to pork chop mixture.

Simmer for 3 hours, stirring occasionally.

Remove pork chops from sauce; discard bones, chop meat, and return to sauce.

Add oregano and thyme the last ½ hour. When mixture is finished cooking, add sugar substitute to taste.

TOTAL GRAMS 120.6
GRAMS PER SERVING 5.0

Green Sauce for Pasta

390 ml

5 cloves garlic, minced
2 tablespoons dried basil
¼ teaspoon dried thyme
25 g grated Parmesan cheese
35 g chopped walnuts
90 ml olive oil
90 g butter
2 tablespoons chopped parsley

Place garlic, basil, thyme, Parmesan cheese, walnuts, and 2 teaspoons of the oil in blender. Blend until smooth. Add remaining oil, 2 tablespoons at a time, and blend. Serve on pasta topped with 15 g butter per serving. Garnish with chopped parsley.

TOTAL GRAMS 10.9
GRAMS PER 15 ML/1 TABLESPOON SERVING 0.4

Mustard Sauce

300 ml

60 ml Dijon mustard
230 g soured cream
2 tablespoons chopped chives

Mix ingredients well. Refrigerate.

TOTAL GRAMS 13.0
GRAMS PER 15 ML/1 TABLESPOON 0.7

Hot Barbecue Sauce

300 ml

30 g butter
1 medium onion, chopped
1 clove garlic, minced
60 ml prepared tomato sauce or passata
30 ml wine vinegar
Tabasco sauce to taste
2 tablespoons sugar substitute
1 teaspoon salt
1 teaspoon dry mustard
60 ml water

Melt butter in saucepan. Sauté onion and garlic until golden. Add remaining ingredients and bring to boil. Store in covered jar and refrigerate.

TOTAL GRAMS 16.7
GRAMS PER 15 ML/1 TABLESPOON 0.8

Lemon Barbecue Sauce

180 ml

1 small clove garlic
½ teaspoon salt
125 ml oil
60 ml lemon juice
2 tablespoons chopped onion
½ teaspoon dried thyme
2 teaspoons sugar substitute (optional)

Mash garlic clove in bowl. Add salt. Mix in oil and add remaining ingredients. Chill to blend flavours.

Excellent on grilled fish.

TOTAL GRAMS 8.8
GRAMS PER 15 ML/1 TABLESPOON 0.7

Cranberry Sauce

8 125-ml servings

280 g fresh cranberries
375 ml water
1 × 11.5 g packet sugar-free lemon or orange jelly crystals
5 tablespoons sugar substitute
30 ml cranberry or orange liqueur
1 teaspoon raspberry flavouring (optional)
pinch salt

Cook cranberries in water over low heat until they pop open. Drain and press through sieve into measuring jug. Add boiling water to make 375 ml liquid.

Dissolve jelly crystals, sugar substitute, liqueur, and flavouring if using, in hot liquid. Add cranberry pulp if desired.

Chill until firm. Slice to serve.

TOTAL GRAMS 48.1
GRAMS PER SERVING 6.0

Cheese Sauce

270 ml

180 ml whipping cream
80 ml water
335 g Cheddar cheese, diced
1 teaspoon Dijon mustard
1 teaspoon salt
½ teaspoon paprika

In top of double boiler combine all ingredients. Simmer slowly over hot water, stirring constantly until smooth.

TOTAL GRAMS 11.9
GRAMS PER 15 ML/1 TABLESPOON   0.7

Parsley Butter Sauce

4 30-ml servings

4 sprigs parsley, chopped (tops only)
1 small clove garlic, chopped fine
120 g unsalted butter, melted
¼ teaspoon Worcestershire sauce

In a frying pan add parsley and garlic to melted butter. Cook for 1 minute over medium heat. Add Worcestershire sauce.
　Serve immediately.
　(If you must reheat this sauce, use very low heat.)

TOTAL GRAMS 2.3
GRAMS PER SERVING 0.6

Joan's Ricotta Sauces

150 ml

For Pork:

125 g ricotta cheese
30 ml olive oil
1–2 teaspoons sugar substitute, to taste
1 teaspoon grated orange zest
¼ teaspoon grated nutmeg
⅛ teaspoon ground cloves
⅛ teaspoon ground cinnamon

Mix all ingredients together. Refrigerate for ½ hour.

TOTAL GRAMS 6.0
GRAMS PER 15 ML/1 TABLESPOON 0.6

For Chicken:

125 g ricotta cheese
½ teaspoon curry powder
¼ teaspoon turmeric
¼ teaspoon ground cumin
2 tablespoons soured cream

Mix ingredients together and refrigerate for ½ hour.

TOTAL GRAMS 6.0
GRAMS PER 15 ML/1 TABLESPOON 0.6

For Fish:

125 g ricotta cheese
30 ml whipping cream
1 teaspoon chopped tarragon
1 teaspoon grated lemon zest
1–2 teaspoons sugar substitute, to taste

Mix all ingredients together and refrigerate for ½ hour.

TOTAL GRAMS 6.7
GRAMS PER 5 ML/1 TABLESPOON 0.7

Tomato Purée

120 ml

10 tomatoes, chopped
½ teaspoon salt

Place tomatoes in a saucepan. Sprinkle with salt. Simmer for ½ hour, uncovered. Strain, mashing pulp through sieve. Cool. Store in refrigerator.

TOTAL GRAMS 53.0
GRAMS PER 15 ML/1 TABLESPOON   6.6

Vinegar- and Sugar-Free Ketchup

600 ml

500 ml Tomato Purée *(above)*
125 ml lemon juice
125 ml water
½ teaspoon salt
1 teaspoon dried oregano
⅛ teaspoon ground cumin
⅛ teaspoon ground nutmeg
⅛ teaspoon pepper
½ teaspoon dry mustard
dash garlic powder

Place all ingredients in a blender or food processor and blend well. Refrigerate.

TOTAL GRAMS 23.6
GRAMS PER 15 ML/1 TABLESPOON   0.6

Desserts

Macadamia Nut Candy

10 candies

25 g thick double cream
4 teaspoons sugar substitute
30 g unsweetened desiccated coconut
10 large macadamia nuts

Mix cream and sweetener. Spoon over coconut and mix well. Allow flavors to blend for 2 minutes. Roll nuts in coconut mixture until well covered. Place on wax paper in freezer for 10 minutes before serving.

To store: Wrap well in greaseproof paper and place in freezer bag.

TOTAL GRAMS 26.4
GRAMS PER SERVING 2.7

Almond Balls

12 balls

¼ teaspoon almond essence
3–4 teaspoons sugar substitute
1 tablespoon desiccated coconut
3 tablespoons almond butter*
1 tablespoon mascarpone cheese

Mix almond essence and 2 teaspoons sugar substitute. Spoon over coconut and mix well. Mix almond butter, cheese and 1–2 teaspoons sugar substitute until fully blended.

Roll into 5-mm balls, roll in coconut, and place in freezer for 10 minutes.

To store: Wrap well in greaseproof paper and store in freezer bag.

TOTAL GRAMS 14.5
GRAMS PER SERVING 1.2

---

*Available at health food stores.

Almond Ball Cookies

12 cookies

1 Almond Balls *recipe (page 189)*
2 tablespoons desiccated coconut

Preheat oven to 170° C (gas 3).

Follow *Almond Balls* recipe, add coconut mixture and additional coconut.

Drop by teaspoonsful on to greased baking tray.

Bake for 10 minutes or until golden brown. Be careful not to burn bottoms.

TOTAL GRAMS 21.5
GRAMS PER SERVING   1.8

Pistachio Popcorn Balls

6 balls

15 g or 300 ml fresh popped corn (from 1 tablespoon kernels)
3 tablespoons roasted pistachio nut butter* (or other nut butter)
1 dozen cold shelled pistachio nuts

Mix all ingredients and form into tablespoon-size balls. Serve.

TOTAL GRAMS 21.1
GRAMS PER SERVING   3.5

Basic Frosting

450 ml

4 tablespoons sugar-free vanilla flavour dessert mix
300 ml whipping cream
60 g mascarpone cheese
60 g ricotta cheese
1 teaspoon vanilla essence

Prepare dessert according to packet instructions in a large bowl, using cream as liquid. Allow to set for 5 minutes.

Add mascarpone, ricotta and vanilla to bowl and whisk together.

Chocolate or butterscotch frosting may be made by substituting appropriate dessert mix flavour.

Use frosting on one of our sponge cakes.

TOTAL GRAMS 33.3
GRAMS PER SERVING   2.7

Cannoli Custard Frosting

450 ml, fills 2 cakes

Follow *Basic Frosting* recipe method and place mixture in freezer until frosting is the consistency of soft custard. May be used as cake frosting, between two cake layers, or enjoyed as a custard.

TOTAL GRAMS 33.3
GRAMS PER SERVING   2.7

Ice Cream

Ice cream is a very important part of this diet. It has long been enjoyed as the special, delicious climax of afternoon picnics, informal lunches and formal dinners. Dr. Atkins has been known to eat it watching football on a Sunday afternoon.

Because we all love it so much, I have perfected seven (one for each day of the week) fail-safe ice cream recipes. Two of the recipes (*Vanilla* and *Coffee*) you may have from the beginning of the diet. *Coconut Macadamia, Butter Pecan,* and *Maple Walnut* may be added to the Ongoing Weight Loss. Premaintenance welcomes *Raspberry Rapture* and *Chocolate*. Maintenance offers *Chunky Chocolate Fudge Ice Cream* plus two frozen yoghurts and two creamy sorbets.

Preparing these creamy delights is easy. All you need are these recipes and an ice cream maker. This may sound expensive but it need not be. Hand-churned ice cream makers are very low in price. Using them is easy. The preparation time is a little longer because the custard must be refrigerated for two hours before you can churn it. The electric machines start at about £30 and go up. The most economical require some available freezer space as the custard is churned in a container you pre-freeze in your freezer. The entire process takes about $\frac{1}{2}$ hour once the prepared custard is cooled or chilled. You will rejoice at the way these ice cream makers make dessert (ice cream) while you eat dinner.

Also available are electric ice cream makers with integral freezer units. These machines are more expensive, but offer the convenience of making ice cream at a moment's notice and the capability of making several batches of ice cream on the trot. Both types of machine make delicious ice creams from these recipes.

Basic Ice Cream Custard

6 125-ml servings

500 ml whipping cream
4 egg yolks
½ vanilla pod, slit open and scraped
5 tablespoons sugar substitute

Heat cream in a heavy saucepan over a low heat. Whisk in one egg yolk at a time. Add vanilla pod scrapings and whisk until custard begins to thicken. Remove from heat and cool. Beat one tablespoon of sugar substitute at a time into cooled custard. At this point the custard is ready to add recipe ingredients that make it ice cream (see recipes that follow). Do not overlook the value of refrigerating the custard as it is and using it as a delicious, rich dessert. Or you could whisk in a tablespoon of brandy or brandy flavouring and serve it over berries. An elegant custard sauce, indeed.

TOTAL GRAMS 20.8
GRAMS PER SERVING 3.5

Chocolate Ice Cream

8 125-ml servings

1 recipe Basic Ice Cream Custard *(above)*
50 g cocoa powder
2 tablespoons sugar substitute
2 tablespoons sugar-free chocolate dessert mix powder (optional)

Prepare *Basic* recipe, above. Whisk in cocoa powder. Beat until smooth. Remove from stove and whisk in sugar substitute and dessert mix powder. Cool to room temperature. Place custard in ice cream maker. Churn according to manufacturer's instructions.

TOTAL GRAMS 58.8
GRAMS PER SERVING 7.4

Chunky Chocolate Fudge Ice Cream

9 125-ml servings

1 recipe Chocolate Ice Cream *(page 193)*
½ recipe Chocolate Fudge *(page 211)*

Prepare *Chocolate Ice Cream* and *Chocolate Fudge* recipes. Cut fudge into 5-mm squares. Add to ice cream maker just before ice cream is ready.

TOTAL GRAMS 72.5
GRAMS PER SERVING 8.0

Raspberry Rapture Ice Cream

8 125-ml servings

1 recipe Basic Ice Cream Custard *(page 193)*
½–1 teaspoon raspberry flavouring, to taste
1 tablespoon Framboise (red raspberry liqueur)
125 g raspberries
2 tablespoons sugar substitute

Prepare *Basic Ice Cream Custard.* Allow to cool.

Mix raspberry flavouring and Framboise together. Place raspberries in a small bowl. Sprinkle with sugar substitute. Add syrup and Framboise. Chill to allow flavours to blend, about 5 minutes.

Whisk raspberry mixture into cooling custard. Cool to room temperature. Place in ice cream maker and churn according to manufacturer's instructions.

TOTAL GRAMS 39.4
GRAMS PER SERVING 4.9

Vanilla Ice Cream

6 125-ml servings

1 recipe Basic Ice Cream Custard *(page 193)*
1 tablespoon vanilla essence

Prepare *Basic Ice Cream Custard*. While cooling, whisk in vanilla essence. Cool to room temperature.

Place in ice cream maker and churn according to manufacturer's instructions.

TOTAL GRAMS 32.2
GRAMS PER SERVING 5.4

Butter Pecan Ice Cream

8 125-ml servings

1 recipe Basic Ice Cream Custard *(page 193)*
30 g unsalted butter
100 g pecan halves, coarsely chopped
1 tablespoon sugar substitute
1 teaspoon butterscotch flavouring (optional)

Prepare *Basic Ice Cream Custard*. Allow to cool.

Melt butter in a small frying pan. Add nuts to pan. Sauté for one minute. Sprinkle with sugar substitute. Remove from heat and mix well, coating nuts completely. Whisk butterscotch flavouring, if using, and nuts into cooling custard mixture. Cool to room temperature. Place in ice cream maker and churn according to manufacturer's instructions.

TOTAL GRAMS 61.2
GRAMS PER SERVING 7.7

Coconut Macadamia Ice Cream

8 125-ml servings

1 recipe Basic Ice Cream Custard *(page 193)*
25 g grated fresh coconut, or unsweetened desiccated coconut
½ teaspoon rum essence or flavouring
70 g whole unsalted macadamia nuts
½ teaspoon vanilla essence
4 teaspoons sugar substitute

Prepare *Basic Ice Cream Custard.* Allow to cool.

Place coconut in a small bowl and sprinkle rum essence on it. Stir to combine flavours. Whisk coconut, macadamia nuts, vanilla essence and sugar substitute into cooling custard. Cool to room temperature. Place in ice cream maker and churn according to manufacturer's instructions.

TOTAL GRAMS 40.8
GRAMS PER SERVING 5.1

Maple Walnut Ice Cream

8 125-ml servings

1 recipe Basic Ice Cream Custard *(page 193)*
1 tablespoon maple or caramel flavouring
30 g unsalted butter
4 teaspoons sugar substitute
120 g walnut halves

Prepare *Basic Ice Cream Custard.* Whisk in maple or caramel flavouring. Melt butter in a small frying pan. Add nuts and sauté for 1 minute. Sprinkle with sugar substitute and mix well. Add nuts to custard and cool to room temperature. Place in ice cream maker and churn according to manufacturer's instructions.

TOTAL GRAMS 34.6
GRAMS PER SERVING 4.3

Decaf-Coffee Ice Cream

8 125-ml servings

1 recipe Basic Ice Cream Custard *(page 193)*
1 cup very strong decaffeinated coffee
1 tablespoon coffee flavouring or liqueur

Prepare *Basic Ice Cream Custard* recipe. Brew coffee by using 2 cups water and 4 tablespoons decaffeinated ground coffee. When brewed, simmer over a low flame until it reduces by half. Remove from heat. Whisk in coffee flavouring or liqueur and allow to cool. Whisk coffee mixture into *Basic Ice Cream Custard.* Cool to room temperature. Place in ice cream maker and churn according to manufacturer's instructions.

TOTAL GRAMS 28.0
GRAMS PER SERVING 3.5

Peach Melba Frozen Yoghurt

8 125 ml servings

450 g low fat vanilla yoghurt
2 egg yolks
3 tablespoons sugar substitute
3 Poached Peaches, *diced (page 215)*
1 teaspoon raspberry flavouring

Whisk yoghurt, egg yolks and sugar substitute together over a low heat. Stir until mixture begins to thicken. Remove from heat. Add peaches and raspberry flavouring. Mix well. Cool to room temperature. Place in ice cream maker and churn according to manufacturer's instructions.

TOTAL GRAMS 65.7
GRAMS PER SERVING 8.2

Chocolate Frozen Yoghurt

4 125-ml servings

450 g low fat vanilla yoghurt
2 egg yolks
4 tablespoons sugar substitute
2 tablespoons cocoa

Heat yoghurt on low heat. Whisk in egg yolks, sugar substitute and cocoa powder. Stir until mixture begins to thicken. Remove from heat and cool to room temperature. Place in ice cream maker and churn according to manufacturer's instructions.

TOTAL GRAMS 65.7
GRAMS PER SERVING 16.4

Raspberry Sorbet

8 120-ml servings

250 ml whipping cream
2 egg yolks
1 teaspoon lemon essence
3 tablespoons sugar substitute
125 g raspberries
1 teaspoon raspberry flavouring
125 ml Framboise (red raspberry liqueur)

Heat cream on low heat. Whisk in egg yolks one at a time. Add lemon extract and 4 packets of sugar substitute. Whisk until mixture begins to thicken. Remove from heat.

Rinse and dry raspberries. Place in a bowl. Sprinkle with sugar substitute. Add raspberry flavouring and Framboise. Mix well.

Whisk raspberry mixture into cream mixture. Cool to room temperature.

Place mixture in ice cream maker and churn according to manufacturer's instructions.

TOTAL GRAMS 37.4
GRAMS PER SERVING 4.7

Grapefruit Sorbet

8 125-ml servings

250 ml whipping cream
2 egg yolks
3 tablespoons sugar substitute
250 ml fresh grapefruit juice
1 × 11.5 g packet sugar-free lemon jelly crystals
125 ml Cointreau (orange liqueur)

Heat cream on low heat. Whisk in one egg yolk at a time. Remove from heat. Whisk in sugar substitute.

Heat grapefruit juice to boiling. Pour over jelly crystals and mix until they are completely dissolved. Whisk in Cointreau. Mix grapefruit mixture with cream. Blend very well. Place in ice cream maker and churn according to manufacturer's instructions.

TOTAL GRAMS 52.7
GRAMS PER SERVING   6.6

Italian Rum Cake

12 servings

1 recipe Lemon Sponge Cake *(page 201)*
1 recipe Cannoli Custard Frosting *(page 191)*
1 tablespoon rum or rum flavouring
1 recipe Chocolate Basic Frosting *(page 191)*

Bake two layers of *Sponge Cake* and cool. Mix rum with *Custard.* Spread custard on top of one cake layer. Add second layer. Cover with *Frosting.*

TOTAL GRAMS 85.7
GRAMS PER SERVING   7.1

Confetti Mould

8 servings

1 × 11.5 g packet sugar-free strawberry jelly crystals
1 × 11.5 g packet sugar-free lime jelly crystals
1 × 11.5 g packet sugar-free orange jelly crystals
3 × 11.5 g packets sugar-free lemon jelly crystals
250 ml whipping cream
1 teaspoon vanilla essence

Prepare first 3 packets of jelly crystals separately, using 375 ml water each. Refrigerate each in separate shallow pans until thoroughly firm. Dice each into tiny cubes.

Mix all 3 packets of lemon jelly crystals with 685 ml water. Allow to thicken. When mixture is very thick, but not firm, add cream. Thicken again. Fold in all flavours of jelly cubes and vanilla essence. Chill until thoroughly firm, in a decorative mould.

TOTAL GRAMS 23.0
GRAMS PER SERVING 2.9

Chocolate Peanut Butter Biscuits

24 biscuits

90 g soy flour
2 teaspoons cocoa powder
1½ teaspoons baking powder
2½ tablespoons sugar substitute
pinch salt
85 g sugar-free peanut butter
1 egg, beaten
1 teaspoon melted butter
125 ml whipping cream
1 teaspoon vanilla essence
½ teaspoon chocolate essence or flavouring

Preheat oven to 190° C (gas 5).

Sift dry ingredients into bowl.

Combine peanut butter with remaining ingredients and add to flour mixture. Stir until blended.

Drop by teaspoonsful on to greased baking tray. Bake for 10–12 minutes until brown.

TOTAL GRAMS 47.9
GRAMS PER BISCUIT   2.0

Lemon Sponge Cake

8 servings

125 ml whipping cream
140 g soy flour
1½ teaspoons baking powder
dash salt
3 eggs
3 tablespoons sugar substitute
2 teaspoons vanilla essence
1 teaspoon lemon essence

Preheat oven to 150° C (gas 2).

Scald cream and remove from heat.

Sift flour, baking powder and salt together.

Whisk eggs and sugar substitute thoroughly until thick and lemon coloured. Blend in flour mixture just until smooth. Add warm cream and essences to mixture. Pour batter immediately into a 23-cm greased tube mould. Bake for 45 minutes, or until done.

TOTAL GRAMS 56.0
GRAMS PER SERVING   7.0

Spice Cake

8 servings

250 ml whipping cream
140 g soy flour
1½ teaspoons baking powder
pinch salt
½ teaspoon ground cinnamon
⅛ teaspoon ground cloves
¼ teaspoon grated nutmeg
3 eggs
3 tablespoons sugar substitute
1 teaspoon brandy flavouring
2 teaspoons vanilla essence

Preheat oven to 170° C (gas 3).

Scald cream and remove from heat. Sift flour, baking powder, salt and spices together.

Whisk eggs with sugar substitute until very thick. Blend in flour mixture until smooth. Add warm cream and flavourings to mixture. Pour batter immediately into 20-cm greased round cake tin. Bake for 40 minutes, or until done.

TOTAL GRAMS 53.7
GRAMS PER SERVING   6.7

Chocolate Sponge Layer Cake

8 servings

70 g soy flour
½ teaspoon baking powder
pinch salt
1 tablespoon cocoa powder
2 eggs
3 tablespoons sugar substitute
1 teaspoon vanilla essence
1 teaspoon chocolate essence

Preheat oven to 170° C (gas 3).

Sift flour, baking powder, salt and cocoa powder together.

Whisk eggs with sugar substitute until very thick.

Stir in essences. Fold in flour mixture. Bake in greased cake tin for 30 minutes or until done. Makes 1 layer.

TOTAL GRAMS 30.9
GRAMS PER SERVING 3.9

Marzipan

24 2.5-cm forms

200 g unsweetened desiccated coconut
1 packet sugar-free jelly crystals (any fruit flavour)
120 g ground almonds
125 ml whipping cream
2½ tablespoons sugar substitute
½ teaspoon vanilla essence
½ teaspoon almond essence

Combine all ingredients. Shape into any designs you like—fruits, vegetables, and so forth. (Food colouring may be added to simulate true details.)

Chill until forms hold their shape.

TOTAL GRAMS 95.3
GRAMS PER SERVING 4.0

Almond Tart Pastry

1 tart case

140 g soy flour
60 g ground almonds
1 tablespoon sugar substitute
pinch ground cinnamon
75 g butter, chilled

Preheat oven to 200° C (gas 6).

Stir first 4 ingredients together. Rub in butter. Work well into dry ingredients.

Cover pastry with greaseproof paper and refrigerate for 1 hour.

Place in pie or tart tin, patting crumb mixture over sides and bottom of tin with back of spoon. Use fork tines to decorate edges of pastry and to prick holes in bottom and sides. Line pastry case with foil and baking beans, or with an empty tart tin (to keep crust from puffing). Bake for 30 minutes until solid and brown around edges. Remove foil and beans or second tin, cover edges with foil, and allow centre to brown thoroughly, about 5 minutes. Cool.

Substitute for *Meringue Tart Case* (page 213) when on Maintenance.

TOTAL GRAMS 42.1

Lemon Chiffon Pie

8 servings

3 egg yolks, beaten
375 ml water
1 tablespoon sugar substitute
1 × 11.5 g packet sugar-free lemon jelly crystals
30 ml lemon juice
1 teaspoon lemon essence
½ teaspoon grated lemon zest
3 egg whites
⅛ teaspoon salt
1 recipe Meringue Tart Case, *baked (page 213)*

Combine egg yolks, 250 ml of the water, and sugar substitute in a saucepan. Simmer, stirring constantly, until mixture begins to boil. Remove from heat, and stir in jelly crystals. Add remainder of water, lemon juice, lemon essence and zest. Chill until somewhat thickened.

Whisk egg whites and salt until mixture stands in stiff peaks. Stir jelly mixture slightly and fold in egg whites. Pour into prepared *Meringue Tart Case.* Chill until firm.

TOTAL GRAMS 27.4
GRAMS PER SERVING 3.4

Coconut Cream Pie

10 servings

45 g desiccated coconut
30 ml Cointreau
15 g butter
625 ml whipping cream
1 tablespoon gelatine
60 ml cold water
4 tablespoons sugar substitute
4 egg whites, at room temperature
2 teaspoons vanilla essence
1 recipe Meringue Tart Case, *baked (optional) (page 213)*

Place coconut in flameproof bowl. Heat Cointreau and ignite. Pour over coconut. (Flames will be high.)

Heat butter in frying pan. Add coconut and lightly toast it. Remove 2 tablespoons toasted coconut and set aside. Add 250 ml of the cream to pan. Simmer 4 minutes.

Sprinkle gelatine over cold water. Mix well to dissolve. Add to cream mixture. Simmer and stir until it begins to thicken. Remove from heat. Add half the sugar substitute. Cool.

Whisk egg whites until stiff with 2 teaspoons of the remaining sugar substitute.

Fold egg whites into cool cream mixture.

Pour mixture into tart or pie tin sprayed with non-stick cooking spray, or into prepared and baked *Meringue Tart Case.*

Refrigerate until firm.

Whip the remaining 375 ml cream with vanilla and remaining sugar substitute. Pile on top of firm cream mixture. Refrigerate for at least 2 hours before serving. Sprinkle with reserved coconut.

TOTAL GRAMS 37.3
GRAMS PER SERVING 3.7

Chocolate Mint Pie

8 servings

75 g chopped pecans or walnuts
1 recipe Meringue Tart Case (page 213), ready to bake
15 g butter
2 tablespoons hot water
35 g cocoa essence
2 tablespoons peppermint essence
1 teaspoon vanilla essence
1 tablespoon crème de cacao liqueur
6 tablespoons sugar substitute, or more to taste
500 ml whipping cream

Preheat oven to 140° C (gas 1).

Sprinkle chopped nuts over *Meringue Tart Case* and bake for 1 hour until lightly browned and crisp to touch. Cool, preferably leaving in oven until cool.

Melt butter in water in double boiler, stir in cocoa and cook until smooth. Remove from heat, and add peppermint and vanilla essences, crème de cacao and sugar substitute.

Whip cream with 2 teaspoons of the sugar substitute. Fold half the whipped cream into chocolate mixture.

Spoon into tart case and chill for 2–3 hours.

Just before serving, spread remaining whipped cream over top.

TOTAL GRAMS 63.4
GRAMS PER SERVING   7.9

Cheesecake

12 servings

450 g full fat soft (cream) cheese, at room temperature
3 eggs
230 g crème fraîche or soured cream
scraped seeds from ½ vanilla pod
8 tablespoons sugar substitute

Preheat oven to 180° C (gas 4).

Place all ingredients in a blender and blend for 15 minutes. Pour mixture into a 23-cm springform tin. Enclose bottom and sides of tin in a single piece of aluminium foil to prevent leaking. Place in a pan of hot water in oven. If water evaporates during baking, add more hot water as needed. Bake for 1 hour, turn off oven and leave cake in oven 1 hour more.

TOTAL GRAMS 33.0
GRAMS PER SERVING 2.8

Coffee Cream Layer Cake

10 servings

5 egg whites, at room temperature
4 tablespoons sugar substitute
500 ml whipping cream
1½ teaspoons instant decaffeinated coffee granules
1½ teaspoons gelatine
1 tablespoon cold water
45 g butter, at room temperature
4 egg yolks, at room temperature
1 teaspoon each coffee and chocolate flavouring
75 g chopped walnuts

Preheat oven to 140° C (gas 1).

Butter 3 round layer cake tins.

Whisk egg whites until they form soft peaks. Add 1 tablespoon sugar substitute and beat until stiff. Divide whites among 3 pans. Bake for 45 minutes.

Combine 250 ml of the cream and instant decaf coffee in top of double boiler. Stir with wire whisk until granules dissolve. Dissolve gelatine in cold water. Add gelatine to coffee mixture and heat just to boiling. Stir constantly with whisk. Remove from heat. Whisk in 4 egg yolks, 1 yolk at a time. Add butter and beat well until melted. Add flavourings and remaining sugar substitute. Put in freezer to cool.

Whip remaining cream until stiff.

When coffee mixture is cool, fold into whipped cream and refrigerate until layers are cooked and cooled. Pile cream between layers of meringue as you would frost a layer cake. Top with cream, making sure to cover sides.

Sprinkle nuts on top and sides. Refrigerate until serving time.

TOTAL GRAMS 30.2
GRAMS PER SERVING 3.0

Lemon-Lime Mousse

8 servings

120 g butter
9 egg yolks
juice of 2 lemons
juice of 2 limes
3 tablespoons sugar substitute
2 teaspoons grated lemon zest
4 egg whites
375 ml whipping cream
1 teaspoon vanilla essence

Melt butter in saucepan over low heat.

Beat in egg yolks, one at a time, with wire whisk. Remove from heat. Add juice from lemons and limes, 2½ tablespoons of the sugar substitute, and lemon rind. Beat well. Cool.

Whisk egg whites with remaining sugar substitute and vanilla essence. Fold into chilled mixture. Refrigerate for at least 2 hours.

TOTAL GRAMS 31.1
GRAMS PER SERVING 3.9

Pumpkin Chiffon

8 servings

1 tablespoon gelatine
½ teaspoon salt
½ teaspoon grated nutmeg
½ teaspoon ground cinnamon
¼ teaspoon ground ginger
125 ml cold water
2 egg yolks, slightly beaten
250 ml whipping cream
270 g cooked, mashed pumpkin
4–5 tablespoons sugar substitute
2 egg whites

Combine gelatine, salt and spices. Add half the water. Stir. Mix egg yolks with cream, remaining water and pumpkin in top of double boiler. Add gelatine mixture. Cook over boiling water for 10 minutes, stirring constantly. Refrigerate until thick as unbeaten egg whites. Stir occasionally. Add sugar substitute to taste.

Whisk egg whites until stiff. Fold chilled pumpkin mixture into egg whites. Be careful not to break down volume of egg whites. Turn into 1.5 litre capacity soufflé dish. Refrigerate.

TOTAL GRAMS 39.9
GRAMS PER SERVING 5.0

Ice Lollies

6 lollies

375 ml sugar-free fruit-flavoured soft drink
30 ml whipping cream
sprinkle of sugar substitute (optional)

Mix all ingredients together.

Fill plastic moulds for 6 ice lollies with mixture. Insert stick if desired. (It is best to do this when lollies are partially frozen.)

Freeze.

TOTAL GRAMS 4.5
GRAMS PER SERVING 0.8

Peanut Butter Cookies

40 cookies

125 g chunk-style, sugar-free peanut butter
185 ml whipping cream
75 g chopped pecans
2 teaspoons vanilla essence
2½ tablespoons sugar substitute
2 tablespoons soy flour
1 teaspoon baking powder

Preheat oven to 190° C (gas 5).
   Spray a baking tray with non-stick cooking spray.
   Mix all ingredients in bowl. Blend well.
   Drop mixture on tray by teaspoonfuls. Bake for about 10 minutes.

TOTAL GRAMS 47.6
GRAMS PER SERVING 1.2

Chocolate Fudge

15 squares

1 × 47 g packet sugar-free chocolate instant pudding/Dessert Mix
2½ tablespoons sugar substitute
125 ml whipping cream
1 tablespoon crème de cacao liqueur
50 g chunk-style, sugar-free peanut butter

Mix all ingredients together except peanut butter. Place over low heat and add peanut butter. Heat until peanut butter melts. Stir until well blended.
   Spray a small baking dish with non-stick cooking spray. Spoon mixture into dish. Refrigerate until firm. Slice into at least 15 squares.

TOTAL GRAMS 56.9
GRAMS PER SQUARE 3.8

Brownies

30 squares

120 g butter, at room temperature
2 eggs
3 tablespoons cocoa
2 tablespoons water
2 teaspoons chocolate flavouring
2 tablespoons soy flour
5 tablespoons sugar substitute
75 g coarsely chopped walnuts
45 ml crème de cacao liqueur

Preheat oven to 180° C (gas 4). Grease a 20-cm cake tin or shallow 1.5 litre capacity baking dish.

Cream butter with electric hand mixer. Add eggs one at a time, beating well. Beat in cocoa, water and flavouring.

Add soy flour and sugar substitute to butter mixture. Mix well and fold in walnuts.

Turn batter into prepared tin and smooth top. Bake 15 minutes. Do not overcook. Remove from oven. Sprinkle crème de cacao over top. Cool. Cut into at least 30 squares.

TOTAL GRAMS 49.0
GRAMS PER SQUARE   1.6

Meringue Tart Case

1 pie shell

4 egg whites
1 teaspoon cream of tartar
pinch of salt
4 teaspoons crème de cacao

Preheat oven to 120° C (gas ³⁄₄).

Place egg whites, cream of tartar and salt in bowl. Whisk until frothy. Gradually add crème de cacao. Continue whisking until whites are stiff, glossy and stand in stiff peaks.

Grease a tart or pie tin. Pour meringue into pie tin and form crust by pressing with back of spoon.

Bake for 1 hour.

TOTAL GRAMS 7.4

How to Whisk Egg Whites for Meringues:

Eggs will whisk better at room temperature, but separate better when cold. The trick is to separate them when cold, then let stand until they reach room temperature.

The best way to whisk egg whites is with an electric hand beater; however, a rotary beater will also do the job.

Poached Peaches

10 peach halves

5 ripe summer peaches, stoned and peeled, cut in halves
3 tablespoons water
1 tablespoon sugar substitute
1 teaspoon almond essence

Place peaches and water in a small pan. Simmer covered for 20 minutes.

Add sugar substitute and almond essence to liquid in pan and swirl to dissolve. If preferred, substitute raspberry flavouring for almond.

Serve hot or refrigerate.

TOTAL GRAMS 49.0
GRAMS PER PEACH HALF 4.9

Tomato Lemon Aspic

4 135-ml servings

185 ml boiling water
1 × 11.5 g packet sugar-free lemon jelly crystals
375 ml spicy tomato or vegetable juice, chilled

Bring water to a boil. Dissolve jelly crystals in water. Cool.

Add tomato or vegetable juice and chill until firm.

TOTAL GRAMS 15.2
GRAMS PER SERVING 3.8

Strawberry-Banana Cream

4 135-ml servings

250 ml water
1 teaspoon banana flavouring, or to taste
1 × 11.5 g packet sugar-free strawberry jelly crystals
185 ml sugar-free strawberry flavoured sparking water
100 ml whipping cream

Heat water to a boil. Add banana flavouring. Pour over jelly crystals and stir to completely dissolve. Cool. Add sparkling water and cream. Whisk until well blended. Refrigerate until firm.

TOTAL GRAMS 2.4
GRAMS PER SERVING 0.6

Beverages

Hot Chocolate

1 serving

80 ml whipping cream
160 ml water
1 teaspoon unsweetened cocoa
2 teaspoons sugar substitute
½ teaspoon vanilla essence

Place all ingredients in saucepan. Heat to boiling point, but do not boil. Stir constantly.
   Serve in mug.

TOTAL GRAMS 5.4

Cappuccino

1 serving

1 recipe Hot Chocolate *(above)*
½ teaspoon instant coffee granules
½ teaspoon brandy essence
1 cinnamon stick

Make *Hot Chocolate.* Add coffee and brandy essence.
   Serve in mug with cinnamon stick.

TOTAL GRAMS 8.1

Spicy Cocktail

2 servings

500 ml Beef Stock *(page 71)*
4 teaspoons prepared tomato sauce
½ teaspoon onion juice or grated onion
½ teaspoon Worcestershire sauce
2 drops Tabasco sauce

Combine all ingredients. Mix well. Serve hot or cold.

TOTAL GRAMS 4.1
GRAMS PER SERVING 2.1

Orange Cooler

4 servings

1 × 11.5 g packet sugar-free orange flavour jelly crystals
2 egg whites, whisked stiffly
2 teaspoons lemon zest, grated
1 teaspoon orange essence
1 tablespoon sugar substitute
4 strawberries
4 ice cubes
4 lemon slices

Prepare jelly according to package directions and cool.

Beat in whisked egg whites with wire whisk. Add lemon zest, orange essence and sugar substitute.

Place in blender. Add strawberries and ice cubes. Blend at medium speed for 30 seconds.

Pour into glasses and garnish with lemon slices.

TOTAL GRAMS 10.2
GRAMS PER SERVING 2.5

Black and White Ice Cream Soda

1 serving

²/₃ glass sugar-free cola (about 165 ml)
30 ml whipping cream
2 scoops Vanilla Ice Cream *(page 195)*

Mix cream into cola. Add *Ice Cream. Serve immediately.*

TOTAL GRAMS 6.0

Blender-Thick Raspberry Shake

2 servings

2 scoops Vanilla Ice Cream *(page 195) or Raspberry Rapture Ice Cream (page 194)*
45 ml whipping cream
1–2 teaspoons raspberry flavouring
250 ml diet ginger ale

Place all ingredients in blender. Blend for 1 minute at medium speed.

TOTAL GRAMS 7.9
GRAMS PER SERVING 4.0

Chocolate Shake

1 serving

1 tablespoon gelatine
250 ml diet cola
1 tablespoon unsweetened cocoa
4 ice cubes
1 teaspoon chocolate essence
80 ml whipping cream
2 teaspoons sugar substitute
dash of salt

Place gelatine, 60 ml of the cola and cocoa in saucepan. Stir well. Heat slowly to boiling point. Be sure gelatine dissolves completely. Cool.

Place ice cubes in blender. Add cooled gelatine mixture, chocolate essence, cream, remaining cola, sugar substitute and salt. Blend at high speed for 30 seconds.

Serve in tall glass. It will become thicker as it sets. Stir vigorously.

TOTAL GRAMS 5.8

Shape-Up Shake

1 serving

1 × 11.5 g packet sugar-free lime jelly crystals
250 ml diet lemon-lime soft drink
4 ice cubes
80 ml whipping cream
2 teaspoons sugar substitute

Place jelly crystals and 60 ml of the soft drink in saucepan. Heat to boiling point, stirring constantly. Be sure jelly crystals dissolve.
Cool.
Place ice cubes in blender, add jelly mixture, cream, remaining soft drink and sugar substitute.
Blend at high speed for 30 seconds.
Serve in tall glass. It will become thicker as it sets. Stir vigorously.

TOTAL GRAMS 3.7

Mocha Drink

1 serving

250 ml brewed decaffeinated coffee
250 ml diet cola
1 teaspoon chocolate essence
4 ice cubes
¼ teaspoon ground cinnamon
30 ml whipping cream
1 organic egg
2 teaspoons sugar substitute (optional)

Place all ingredients in a blender and blend until smooth.

TOTAL GRAMS 3.9

Spiced Iced Decaf Coffee

4 servings

2 tablespoons decaffeinated instant coffee granules
5 whole allspice
5 whole cloves
dash cinnamon
750 ml boiling water
8 ice cubes
4 teaspoons whipping cream

Combine all ingredients except cream in a 1-litre container. Cover and refrigerate 1 hour or more.

Strain. Pour over ice cubes into 4 tall glasses.

Add 1 teaspoon cream to each glass.

TOTAL GRAMS 3.8
GRAMS PER SERVING 1.0

Still Lemonade with Lecithin

4 servings

250 ml water
60 ml lemon juice
3–4 teaspoons sugar substitute
2 egg whites
1 teaspoon vanilla essence
½ teaspoon orange essence
dash salt
8 ice cubes
2 teaspoons lecithin

Place all ingredients except ice cubes and lecithin in a blender. Blend until thick.

Add 1 ice cube at a time and blend until frothy.

Remove from blender and stir in lecithin. Pour into 4 glasses. Stir again and serve immediately.

TOTAL GRAMS 21.7
GRAMS PER SERVING   5.4

Hot Mint Chocolate Nog

1 serving

250 ml peppermint tea
1 teaspoon chocolate essence or flavouring
1 tablespoon sugar substitute
1 organic egg
30 ml whipping cream

Place all ingredients in blender. Blend well.

TOTAL GRAMS 4.4

Appendices

Special Menus for Entertaining

FORMAL DINNER

Serves 12

HORS D'OEUVRES

Fran's Special Pâté
Devilled-Salmon Eggs
Caribbean Crab Balls

APPETIZER

Honeydew and Seafood

SOUP

Cold Avocado Soup

SALAD

Tricolour Salad with Three Cheeses

MAIN COURSE

Stuffed Steak
or
Stuffed Flounder

VEGETABLES

Cauliflower Bake
Cheesy Brussels Sprouts

TO CLEAR THE PALATE

Small scoop of Grapefruit Sorbet

DESSERT

Spice Cake with Coconut Macadamia Ice Cream

BEVERAGES

Cappuccino
tea
decaffeinated coffee with cream and sugar substitute

BARBECUE

Serves 12

WHEN FOLKS ARRIVE

Guacamole with cucumber slices
Soured Cream Clam Dip with pork rinds
cheese tray

ON THE COALS

Dr. Atkins Fromage Burgers
Luscious Lamb
Tarragon Lobster Tails (barbecued instead of grilled)
chicken marinated in Hot Barbecue Sauce

THE SALADS

Coleslaw
Mock Potato Salad

SWEETS

Confetti Mould
Decaf-Coffee Ice Cream
Almond Ball Cookies
Chocolate Sponge Layer Cake

DRINKS

Spicy Cocktail
Still Lemonade with Lecithin
Orange Cooler

BUFFET DINNER

Serves 20

APPETIZING TABLE

Fresh Spring Salmon Mousse
Spicy Spare Ribs
Heavenly Wings
Salad Niçoise with Fresh Tuna
assorted olives

ENTRÉE TABLE

Kayzie's Rabbit
Moussaka
Prawns and Scallops Marc
Coq Au Vin with Shiitake Mushrooms

DESSERT TABLE

Lemon-Lime Mousse
Chocolate Mint Pie
Cheesecake
Raspberry Rapture Ice Cream

CANDY TRAY

Almond Balls
Chocolate Fudge
Pistachio Popcorn Balls

BEVERAGES

Cappuccino
tea
decaffeinated coffee with cream and sugar substitute

DESSERT BUFFET ATKINS STYLE

Serves 12

2 CAKES

Italian Rum Cake
Coffee Cream Layer Cake

2 PIES

Coconut Cream Pie
Lemon Chiffon Pie

3 KINDS OF SWEETS

Chocolate Peanut Butter Biscuits
Pistachio Popcorn Balls
Brownies

2 FLAVOURS OF ICE CREAM

Butter Pecan Ice Cream
Chocolate Ice Cream

BEVERAGES

Spiced Iced Tea
Cappuccino
Hot Chocolate

Nutritional Supplementation

Twenty years ago I was almost a voice crying in the wilderness when I said you'd live a longer and healthier life if you ate a healthy diet *and* consumed vitamin and mineral supplements than you would if you ate a healthy diet alone. I have stubbornly persisted because the experiences of my forty thousand patients have affirmed and reaffirmed the correctness of that view. Now the virtues of supplements are becoming commonplace, supported by an increasing number of highly orthodox medical scientists and loudly proclaimed from the covers of major newsmagazines. In the end my viewpoint may become the conventional one, which would be a change of pace.

For all of you who are doing the Atkins diet I must insist on the importance of your supplements. During the two-week Induction phase of the diet, you will need supplements to maintain a proper nutritional balance. After that, you should go right on taking them because they're good for you.

Following is my Dieter's Formula. Find a multivitamin that gives you something close to this formula, and then take three capsules a day. People who weigh 90 kilos or more are to use the second, larger doses, provided in parentheses, of certain vitamins.

Dieter's Formula

Vitamin A	200 IU
Beta-Carotene	500 IU
Vitamin D-2	15 IU
Thiamine (HC1)(B_1)	5 mg
Riboflavin (B_2)	4 mg
Vitamin C (Calcium Ascorbate)	120 mg (150 mg)
Niacin (B_3)	2 mg
Niacinamide	5 mg
Pantethine (80%)	25 mg (30 mg)
Calcium Pantothenate (B_5)	25 mg
Pyridoxal-5-Phosphate	2 mg
Pyridoxine (HCl)(B_6)	20 mg
Folic Acid	100 mcg
Biotin	75 mcg
Cyanocobalamin (B_{12})	30 mcg
Vitamin E (D alpha tocopherol)	2 IU
Copper (Sulfate)	200 mcg
Magnesium (Oxide)	8 mg
Chlorine (Bitartrate)	100 mg
Inositol	80 mg
PABA	100 mg
Manganese (Chelate)	4 mg
Zinc (Chelate)	10 mg
Citrus Bioflavonoids	150 mg
Chromium (Picolinate)	50 mcg
Molybdenum (Sodium)	10 mcg
Vanadyl Sulfate	15 mcg
Selenium	40 mcg
Octacosanol	150 mcg
N-Acetyl-1-cysteine	20 mg
L-Glutathione (reduced)	5 mg

The recommended formula comes in a base of lactobacillus, bulgaris and bifidus acidophilus, B-Complex, and growth factors.

In addition to this formula, the next most important nutritional group for long-range supplementation are the essential fatty acids. You won't find these in a multivitamin formula because they exist physically as oils and don't mix with a dry powder capsule. There are two types of essential fatty acids that most of us need. One type is the omega-3 series that provides you with alpha linolenic acid (ALA). The other type is the omega-6 series called gamma linolenic acid (GLA).

To supplement with these important nutrients, take an essential oils formula containing approximately the following:

Flaxseed oil	400 mg
Borage oil	400 mg
Super EPA	400 mg

Carbohydrate Gram Counter

Foods	*Grams of Carbohydrate*

CONDIMENTS

Anchovies (30 g)	0.0
Cocoa powder, unsweetened (6 g)	2.8
Horseradish (5 ml)	0.5
Mayonnaise (14 g)	0.4
Mustard:	
Dijon (5 g)	0.3
English (5 g)	0.3
Pickles, dill (60 g)	1.4
Soy sauce (15 ml)	2.0
Vinegar:	
balsamic (15 ml)	3.0
cider (15 ml)	0.9
tarragon (15 ml)	0.9
wine (15 ml)	0.9
Worcestershire sauce (15 ml)	2.7

DAIRY PRODUCTS

Butter (125 g)	0.0
Cheese:	
Boursin (30 g)	0.1
Brie (30 g)	0.3
Camembert (30 g)	0.1
Cheddar (30 g)	0.4
cottage, creamed (200 g)	5.6
cream/soft cheese (30 g)	0.8
feta (30 g)	1.2
fontina (30 g)	0.4
goat (30 g)	1.0
Jarlsberg (30 g)	1.0
mascarpone (30 g)	0.5
mozzarella (30 g)	0.6

Foods	**Grams of Carbohydrate**

DAIRY PRODUCTS *(continued)*
Cheese (continued):

muenster (30 g)	0.3
Parmesan (30 g)	0.4
provolone (30 g)	0.6
ricotta (30 g)	1.0
Roquefort (30 g)	0.6
Swiss (30 g)	1.0

Cream:

double/whipping (30 g)	2.0
single (30 g)	0.8
soured (30 g)	1.0
whipped (30 g)	0.8
Milk (full fat, 125 ml)	11.4

Yoghurt, plain:

full fat (225 g)	10.6
Greek style (225 g)	15.6
low fat (225 g)	15.0

FATS/OILS

Groundnut	0.0–trace
Olive	0.0–trace
Rapeseed	0.0–trace
Sunflower	0.0–trace
Walnut	0.0–trace

FRUIT

Apple, medium (135 g flesh)	21.1
Apple sauce, unsweetened (125 g)	13.8
Apricots (3 fresh)	11.8

Avocado:

Fuerte	12.0
Hass	27.1
Banana (1 medium)	26.7
Blackberries (145 g)	18.4

Foods	**Grams of Carbohydrate**

FRUIT (continued)

Blueberries (145 g)	20.5
Cantaloupe (160 g flesh)	13.4
Cherries (70 g raw, sweet)	11.2
Cranberries (100 g)	11.0
Grapefruit (½, pink)	9.5
Grapefruit juice (125 ml)	11.2
Grapes (80 g)	15.8
Honeydew (80 g)	7.7
Kiwi (1 medium)	11.3
Lemon (1 medium)	5.4
Lemon juice (15 ml, fresh)	1.3
Lemon zest (5 ml)	0.3
Lime juice (30 ml)	2.8
Mango (½ medium)	17.1
Olives:	
black (10 olives)	3.0
green, stoned	0.5
Orange (1 medium)	16.3
Orange zest (5 ml)	0.5
Papaya (⅓ medium)	9.9
Peach (90 g, stoned)	9.7
Pear (165 g)	25.1
Pineapple (155 g)	19.2
Plum (1 medium)	8.6
Poached peaches, unsweetened (160 g)	20.0
Prunes, cooked (100 g)	29.8
Raspberries (125 g)	14.2
Rhubarb (120 g, raw)	3.5
Strawberries (150 g)	10.5

GELATINE

Gelatine	0.0
Sugar-free jelly crystals (all flavours, made up, per serving)	0.2

Foods	**Grams of Carbohydrate**

GRAINS

Bagel (1) (approx. 55 g)	30.9
Bread:	
rye (1 slice)	12.0
wholemeal (1 slice)	11.4
Noodles (cooked, 160 g)	37.3
Polenta (cooked, 230 g)	25.7
Popcorn (popped, 10 g)	4.6
Porridge oats (cooked, 240 g)	27.8
Rice:	
white, cooked (200 g)	49.6
puffed (20 g, dry)	19.0
Soya flour (90 g)	27.1

HERBS AND SPICES

Allspice (ground, 15 ml)	1.4
Basil (dried, 15 ml)	0.9
Caraway (seeds, 15 ml)	1.1
Celery (seeds, 15 ml)	0.8
Cinnamon (ground, 15 ml)	1.8
Curry powder (15 ml)	1.0
Dill (15 ml)	1.2
Garlic clove (1)	1.0
Ginger root:	
fresh (30 g)	3.6
ground (5 ml)	1.3
Saffron (5 ml)	0.5
Tarragon (dried, 15 ml)	0.8
Thyme (dried, 15 ml)	0.4
Vanilla, extract or essence (15 ml)	3.0

Foods   **Grams of**
                                                               Carbohydrate

NUTS AND SEEDS

Almond paste (unsweetened, 30 g)	12.4
Almonds:	
shelled, 30 g	5.8
12–15 nuts	2.9
Brazil (4 nuts)	1.8
Cashews (30 g)	9.3
Coconut (fresh, 1 piece 5x5x1 cm)	6.9
Grated coconut, unsweetened desiccated (30 g)	6.7
Hazelnuts (30 g)	5.0
Macadamia nuts (6 nuts)	3.9
Mixed (8–12 nuts, roasted)	6.1
Peanut butter:	
regular (30 g) (average of several brands)	4.0–7.0
sugar-free (30 g) (average of several brands)	3.0
Peanuts (dry roasted, 30 g)	6.0
Pecans (10 halves)	3.5
Pine kernels (30 g)	4.0
Pistachio (30 nuts, roasted)	4.5
Pumpkin seeds (30 g/142 seeds, dried/roasted)	5.1/3.8
Sesame seeds (30 g)	7.0
Soy beans, roasted (30 g)	10.1
Sunflower seeds (30 g, dried, roasted)	5.3
Walnuts (8–10 halves)	6.7
Water chestnuts (30 g)	7.4

PROTEIN (LEAN, WITHOUT SKIN OR BREADING)

Eggs	0.6
Egg yolk	0.0–trace
Egg white	0.0–trace
Fish	0.0–trace
Meat	0.0–trace
Poultry	0.0–trace
Tofu (100g), raw, firm	5.4

Foods	**Grams of Carbohydrate**

PULSES (COOKED)

Black-eyed peas (165 g)	35.5
Butterbeans (60 g)	16.0/21.2
Haricot (190 g), dried, boiled	47.9
Peanuts (60 g), oil or dry roasted	9.8/12.0
Red kidney (80 g)	20.2
Soy beans (90 g), green, boiled	10.0
Split peas (200 g), boiled	41.4
Tofu (100 g), raw, firm	5.4

SOUPS

Chicken Consommé (250 ml)	1.8
Clam Stock (30 ml)	0.6
Cream of Chicken (250 ml)	9.3
Cream of Mushroom (250 ml)	9.3
Minestrone (250 ml)	11.2
Turkey Rice (250 ml)	7.2
Vegetable, creamy (250 ml)	15.0/19.0

VEGETABLES

Asparagus (6 spears)	4.0
Aubergine (diced, 100 g)	6.4
Bamboo shoots (130 g)	4.2
Bean sprouts (100 g)	6.2
Beans:	
green, stringless (60 g, boiled)	4.9
yellow (60 g, boiled)	3.7
Broccoli (steamed, 80 g)	4.3
Brussels sprouts (4, or 80 g)	6.8
Cabbage (raw, shredded, 35 g)	1.9
Carrot (raw, 18 cm)	7.3
Cauliflower (cooked, 125 g)	
Celery (stick, 20 cm long)	1.5
Chicory (25 g)	.8
Chinese leaves (80 g)	3.0
Coleslaw (120 g homemade)	15.0

Foods	**Grams of Carbohydrate**
VEGETABLES (continued)	
Courgette (cooked, 180 g)	8.0
Cucumber (6 slices, 30 g)	1.5
Kale (cooked, 65 g)	3.7
Kohlrabi (cooked, 60 g)	5.5
Lettuce:	
Round (2 leaves)	.4
Iceberg (1 leaf)	.4
Cos/Romaine (2 leaves)	.7
Mushrooms:	
cup (10 small or 4 large, 35 g pieces)	1.6
porcini (70 g)	4.0
shiitake (cooked, 60 g)	10.3
Okra (90 g slices)	5.8
Onion (80 g)	5.9
Pak choi (170 g, cooked)	3.0
Parsley (fresh, 15 ml/2.3 g)	0.3
Parsnips (80 g, boiled)	1.9/15.2
Peas (cooked, 80 g)	25.0
Peppers:	
green (2 rings)	1.4
red (dried, 30 g)	5.0
Potato, baked (flesh, 110 g)	21.0
Potato salad (125 g)	14.0
Pumpkin, fresh (mashed, boiled, 125 g)	6.0
Radish (4 medium)	0.5
Runner beans (60 g)	5.9
Spring onions (6)	2.0
Spinach (cooked, 90 g)	3.4
Squash:	
summer (cooked, 80 g)	3.5
winter (baked, 100 g)	8.9
Swede (1 cup)	13.2
Sweetcorn (1 ear, 80 g)	28.7
Sweet potato (12.5 x 5 cm, baked)	30.0
Tomato:	
cooked, tinned (180 g)	6.8
juice (125 ml)	5.1

Foods	**Grams of Carbohydrate**

VEGETABLES (continued)
Tomato (continued):

purée (30 g)	5.7
raw (120 g)	5.3
sauce, prepared (30 ml)	2.2
sun-dried (average)	2.0–5.0

Turnips:

cooked (150 g)	7.6
greens (150 g, chopped, cooked)	6.2
Vegetable juice (150 ml)	7.0

SAMPLES OF CARBOHYDRATE-RICH "FATTENING" ITEMS

Apple pie (1 slice, homemade)	61.0
Apple pastry	31.1
Banana split	91.0
Blueberry Muffin (1 average)	17.0
Bread stuffing (170 g)	69.0
Brownie (1 average homemade, frosted)	12.7
Cheeseburger ("¼ pounder")	33.0
Donut (1 glazed)	22.0
Egg or spring roll (1)	30.0
French toast (2 slices)	34.0
Fried fish sandwich on roll	64.0
Hot dog with roll (1)	24.0
Ice cream soda (250 ml)	49.0
Ice lolly	17.0
Jam (1 tablespoon/15 ml)	15.0
Macaroni cheese (130 g)	40.0
Onion rings (fast food order)	33.5
Pancake (1 thick)	15.0
Pecan pie (1 piece, homemade)	41.0
Pizza (1 slice)	39.1
Roast beef sandwich	38.8
Shake (medium) average range	46–65
Sherbet (125 ml lemon)	45.0
Taco, beef	14.0

Foods	*Grams of Carbohydrate*

SAMPLES OF CARBOHYDRATE-RICH
"FATTENING" ITEMS (continued)

Tapioca, cream (125 ml)	22.0
Vanilla shake (1 average)	50.8
Waffles (1 homemade, plain)	45.0

Index

Almond Balls, 189
Almond Ball Cookies, 190
Almond Tart Pastry, 203–204
Almond Stuffing, 133
anchovies:
  Salad Niçoise, 89–90
appetizers, 58–67
  Caribbean Crab Balls, 66–67
  Cheesy Ham Snack, 66
  Devilled-Salmon Eggs, 59
  Fran's Special Pâté, 65
  Guacamole, 64
  Heavenly Wings, 62
  Klara's Aubergine Appetizer, 67
  Marbled Tea Eggs From China, 58
  Salami and Parmesan, 62
  Sardine Snack, 63
  Soured Cream Clam Dip, 63
  Swedish Meatballs, 60
  Toasted Nuts, 68
  Turkey Meatballs, 61
  See also salads; salad dressings;
    soups
artichokes:
  Chicken Salad, 85–86
  Green Bean Chokes, 179
  Ham and Artichoke Omelet, 56
asparagus:
  Chic Asparagus, 178
Atkins diet:
  and carbohydrates, 10
  characteristics of, 5

exercise and, 17
foods to avoid, 3, 17
fundamentals of, 5–8
ketosis/lipolysis, 5–7, 10, 14
  ketone bodies, 6
  testing for, 7
and kidney disease, 9
metabolic edge of, 5, 6–7
no hunger diet, 7
nutritional supplementation, 7–8,
  17, 226–227
and pregnant women, 9
preparing for, 8
stages of, 9
  the Induction Diet, 9–14, 17
    allowed foods for, 11–13
    carbohydrate restriction
      during, 10–11
    forbidden foods, 11, 13, 14
    meal plans for, 20–25
    mistakes to avoid, 14
  the rules of, 10–11
    vitamins and, 10
  the Maintenance Diet, 4, 9, 16–18,
    42
  the Ongoing Weight-Loss Diet, 9,
    14–16
    meal plans for, 26–30
  the Premaintenance Diet, 9, 16
    meal plans for, 31–36
  the Yeast-Free Diet, 15, 43
    forbidden foods, 36

meal plans for, 37–41
versus traditional diets, 1–8
Aubergine:
Cheese-Stuffed Aubergine, 170
Aubergine and Cheddar Omelette, 50
Aubergine "Little Shoes", 169–170
Aubergine Parmigiana, 164
Klara's Aubergine Appetizer, 67
Moussaka, 109–110
Ratatouille, 173
Austrian Paprika Chicken, 129
avocados:
Cold Avocado Soup, 75
Crunchy Seafood Salad, 90
Fresh Tuna and Avocado Salad, 80
Guacamole, 64
Not Just Another Tossed Salad, 83
Poached Salmon Salad, 86

bacon:
Bacon and Onion Omelette, 48
Cauliflower Bake, 176
Coq Au Vin with Shiitake Mushrooms, 126
Creamy Ricotta Soup, 73
Fran's Special Pâté, 65
Halibut Roll-Ups, 143
Irene's Turnips, 178
My Grandmother's Veal Stew, 115
New England Clam Chowder, 77
New England Fish Chowder, 76
Not Just Another Tossed Salad, 83
Roast Veal, 113
Baked Scallop and Fish Soup, 77
Baked Spinach, 165
barbecue sauces. See sauces
Basic French Dressing, 95
Basic Frosting, 191
Basic Fried Green Tomatoes, 174
Basic Ice Cream Custard, 193
Basic Omelette, 48
Basic Vinegar-Free Salad Dressing, 93
beans:
Green Bean Chokes, 179
Green Beans Amandine, 167
beef:
Aubergine Little Shoes, 169–70
Beef Stock, 71
Brit Burgers, 104

Cabbage Rolls Stuffed with Meat (Dolma), 120
Calf's Liver in Red Wine, 110
Curry Burgers, 106
Dr. Atkins Fromage Burger, 103
Feta Burgers, 105
Garden Beef, 116
hamburgers, 103–107
Hot Beef Salad, 87
Mother's Pot Roast, 102
Moussaka, 109–110
¡Ole! Burgers, 106
Oriental Beef Stir Fry, 100
Pasta Sauce, 179–180
Pizza Burgers, 104–105
Spicy Spare Ribs, 121
Steak Au Poivre, 108
Steak Pizzaiola, 119
Stuffed Steak, 122
U.S. Hamburgers, 107
beverages, 217–223
Black and White Ice Cream Soda, 219
Blender-Thick Raspberry Shake, 219
Cappuccino, 217
Chocolate Shake, 220
Hot Chocolate, 217
Hot Mint Chocolate Nog, 223
Mocha Drink, 221
Orange Cooler, 218
Shape-Up Shake, 221
Spiced Iced Decaf Coffee, 222
Spicy Cocktail, 218
Still Lemonade with Lecithin, 223
biscuits. see cookies and biscuits
Black and White Ice Cream Soda, 219
Blender-Thick Raspberry Shake, 219
breads, 161–163
4 Grain and Seed Bread, 161
Courgette Bread, 163
Rye Bread, 162
Brit Burgers, 104
broccoli:
Broccoli with Cheese Sauce, 165
Oriental Chicken with Broccoli Rabe, 137–138
Brownies, 212
brussels sprouts:

Cheesy Brussels Sprouts, 177
Butter Pecan Ice Cream, 195

cabbage:
Cabbage Rolls Stuffed with Meat
(Dolma), 120
Coleslaw, 80
Crazy Cabbage, 172
Oriental Prawns, 150
cakes:
Basic Frosting, 191
Brownies, 212
Cannoli Custard Frosting, 191
Cheesecake, 207
Chocolate Sponge Layer Cake,
202–203
Coffee Cream Layer Cake, 208
Italian Rum Cake, 199
Spice Cake, 202
Calf's Liver in Red Wine, 110
candy:
Almond Balls, 189
Chocolate Fudge, 211
Macadamia Nut Candy, 189
Marzipan, 203
Cannelloni, 160
Cannoli Custard Frosting, 191
Cappuccino, 217
carbohydrates, 3, 4
basis of overweight, 3
daily intake of, 4, 6, 7, 9–10
sensitivity to, 3–4
Caribbean Crab Balls, 66–67
cauliflower:
Cauliflower Bake, 176
Cauliflower Cheese Dumplings, 168
Cauliflower Soup with Dill and
Caraway, 78
cheese, recipes featuring:
Aubergine and Cheddar Omelette,
50
Aubergine Parmigiana, 164
Basic Frosting, 187–188
Broccoli in Cheese Sauce, 165
Cannelloni, 160
Cauliflower Cheese Dumplings, 168
Cauliflower with Dill and Caraway,
78
Cheese Sauce, 186
Cheese-Baked Eggs, 47

Cheesecake, 207
Cheese Sauce, 180
Cheese-Stuffed Aubergine, 170
Cheese-Tease Omelette, 49
Cheesy Brussels Sprouts, 177
Cheesy Ham Snack, 66
Chic Asparagus, 178
Crab and Almond Pie, 153
Creamy Ricotta Soup, 73
Dr. Atkins Fromage Burger, 103
Eggs Florentine, 51
Feta Burgers, 105
Fran's Special Pâté, 65
Gnocchi, 157
Goat Cheesy Chicken Rolls, 137
Greek Salad, 84
Ham and Artichoke Omelette, 56
Herb Omelette, 51
Hot Beef Salad, 87
Ivan's Crisp Chicken, 139
Joan's Chicken Mascarpone,
135
Luncheon Omelette, 54
Manicotti, 156
Moulded Roquefort Spread, 81
Not Just Another Tossed Salad, 83
Our Favourite Roquefort Dressing,
95
Parmesan Caesar Dressing, 99
Pizza Burgers, 104–105
Porcini Mushrooms, 175
Prawn and Goat Cheese Omelette,
57
Prawns and Scallops Marc, 152
Prawns Parmesan, 151
Salami and Parmesan, 62
Snappy Swordfish, 141
Spicy Sausage Bake, 53
Tricolour Salad with Three Cheeses,
90
Turkey Meatballs, 61
Two-Cheese Omelette, 55
Veal Rolatine, 111
Veal Scallopini, 114
Chic Asparagus, 178
chicken:
Austrian Paprika Chicken, 129
Cannelloni, 160
Chicken à la Firenze, 127
Chicken Cacciatore, 124

Chicken Croquettes, 130
Chicken Salad, 85–86
Chicken Salad Ham Rolls, 79
Chicken Stock, 69
Coq Au Vin with Shiitake
   Mushrooms, 126
Cream of Chicken Soup, 70
Fran's Special Pâté, 65
Goat Cheesy Chicken Rolls, 137
Gourmet Poussins, 131
Hal's Chicken, 134–135
Heavenly Wings, 62
Ivan's Crisp Chicken, 139
Japanese Egg Custard Soup, 75–76
Joan's Chicken Mascarpone,
   135
Lemon-Basted Roast Chicken, 125
Oriental Chicken with Broccoli
   Rabe, 137–138
Summer Day Chicken From Spain,
   128
Tandoori Chicken, 136
Chinese Mangetout, 169
Chocolate Frozen Yoghurt, 198
Chocolate Fudge, 211
Chocolate Ice Cream, 193
Chocolate Mint Pie, 206
Chocolate Peanut Butter Biscuits,
   200–201
Chocolate Shake, 220
Chocolate Sponge Layer Cake, 202
Chunky Chocolate Fudge Ice Cream,
   194
clams:
   New England Clam Chowder, 77
Coconut Cream Pie, 205
Coconut Macadamia Ice Cream, 196
Cocktail Sauce, 182
cod:
   Baked Scallop and Fish Soup, 77
   New England Fish Chowder, 76
Coffee Cream Layer Cake, 208
Cold Avocado Soup, 75
Coleslaw, 80
Confetti Mould, 200
cookies and biscuits:
   Almond Ball Cookies, 190
   Chocolate Peanut Butter Cookies,
      200
   Peanut Butter Cookies, 211

Coq Au Vin with Shiitake
   Mushrooms, 126
courgette:
   Courgette Bread, 163
   Stuffed Courgettes with Prosciutto,
      166–167
crab:
   Caribbean Crab Balls, 66–67
   Crab and Almond Pie, 153
   Crab and Mushroom Omelette, 55
   Crunchy Seafood Salad, 90
   Curried Crab, 154
Cranberry Sauce, 185
Crazy Cabbage, 172
Cream of Shiitake Mushroom Soup,
   72–73
Cream Sauce, 180
Creamy Celery Seed Dressing, 97
Creamy Ricotta Soup, 73
Crispy White Radish, 176
Crunchy Seafood Salad, 90
cucumbers:
   The Most Delicious Cucumbers,
      171
Curried Crab, 154
Curry Burgers, 106
Curry Dressing, 98

Decaf-Coffee Ice Cream, 197
desserts, 189–216
   Brownies, 212
   Confetti Mould, 200
   Ice Lollies, 210
   Lemon-Lime Mousse, 209
   Marzipan, 203
   Pistachio Popcorn Balls, 190
   Poached Peaches, 215
   See also cakes; candy; cookies; ice
      cream and sorbets; pies; yoghurt
Deviled-Salmon Eggs, 59
Dill Vinaigrette Dressing, 98
Dr. Atkins Fromage Burger, 103
Dr. Atkins New Diet Revolution, 4, 9,
   15
Dressing of the House, 96
duck:
   Duck in Red Wine, 134
Dumpling Soup, 72

egg recipes, 44–59

basics of, 44
Cheese-Baked Eggs, 47
Deviled-Salmon Eggs, 59
Eggs Florentine, 51
Hard-Boiled Eggs, 45
Japanese Egg Custard Soup, 75–76
Marbled Tea Eggs, 58
Mock Potato Salad, 81–82
omelettes:
    Aubergine and Cheddar
        Omelette, 50
    Bacon and Onion Omelette, 48
    Basic Omelette, 48
    Cheese-Tease Omelette, 49
    Crab and Mushroom Omelette,
        55
    Ham and Artichoke Omelette,
        56
    Herb Omelette, 51
    Luncheon Omelette, 54
    Peaches and Cream Omelette,
        49–50
    Prawn and Goat Cheese Omelette,
        57
    Spicy Sausage Bake, 53
    Two-Cheese Omelette, 55
Over Easy, 46
Poached Eggs, 47
Salad Niçoise, 89–90
Salmon Soufflé, 52
Scrambled Eggs, 46
Soft-Boiled Eggs, 45
Sunny-Side Up, 46
Enchiladas, 158

fat, body, 7
fats, dietary, 3, 4, 18
Fennel Red Mullet, 146
Feta Burgers, 105
fish and shellfish recipes, 137–151
    Caribbean Crab Balls, 66–67
    Crab and Almond Pie, 153
    Crab and Mushroom Omelette, 55
    Curried Crab, 154
    Deviled-Salmon Eggs, 59
    Fennel Red Mullet, 146
    Fish Stock, 71
    Fresh Spring Salmon Mousse, 148
    Fresh Tuna and Avocado Salad, 80
    Halibut Roll-Ups, 143

Houston's Ceviche, 155
New England Clam Chowder, 77
New England Fish Chowder, 76
Oriental Prawns, 150
Poached Fish Fillets, 142
Prawn and Goat Cheese Omelette,
    57
Prawns and Scallops Marc, 152
Prawns Parmesan, 151
Salmon Soufflé, 52
Sardine Snack, 63
Snappy Swordfish, 141
Sole with Soured Cream, 144
Soured Cream Clam Dip, 63
Stuffed Sole, 145
Sun Luck Scallops, 140
Tarragon Lobster Tails, 152–153
Trout in Tomato Sauce, 147
Tuna Loaf, 149
4 Grain and Seed Bread, 161
Fran's Special Pâté, 65
French Dressing, Basic, 95
Fresh Spring Salmon Mousse, 148
Fresh Tuna and Avocado Salad, 80
Frozen Horseradish Cream, 180
fruit, recipes featuring:
    Honeydew and Seafood, 85
    Lime Dill Dressing, 92
    Peaches and Cream Omelette,
        49–50
    Peach Melba Frozen Yoghurt, 197
    Poached Peaches, 212

Garden Beef, 116
Gazpacho, 74
Gnocchi, 157
Goat Cheesy Chicken Rolls, 137
Gourmet Pork Chops, 112
Gourmet Poussins, 131
Grapefruit Sorbet, 199
Greek Salad, 84
Green Beans Amandine, 167
Green Bean Chokes, 179
Green Sauce for Pasta, 183
Guacamole, 64

Halibut Roll-Ups, 143
Hal's Chicken, 134–135
ham:
    Almond Stuffing, 133

Baked Spinach, 165
Cannelloni, 160
Cheesy Ham Snack, 66
Chicken Salad Ham Rolls, 79
Ham and Artichoke Omelette, 56
Oriental Prawns, 150
Stuffed Courgettes with Prosciutto, 166–167
Stuffed Steak, 122
Veal Rolatine, 111
hamburgers, 103–107
Hard-Boiled Eggs, 45
health problems, 3
  allergies, 3
  blood-pressure checks, 3
  blood sugar levels and, 3, 4, 18
  blood tests for, 3
  cholesterol levels, 3
  diabetes, 3
  fatigue and irritability, 3
  heart disease, 3, 18
  hypertension, 3
  insulin levels and, 3, 4, 18
  yeast infections, 15
Heavenly Wings, 62
Herb Omelette, 51
Hollandaise Sauce, 181
Honeydew and Seafood, 85
Hot Barbecue Sauce, 184
Hot Beef Salad, 87
Hot Chocolate, 217
Hot Mint Chocolate Nog, 223
Houston's Ceviche, 155

ice cream and sorbets, 192–199
  Basic Ice Cream Custard, 193
  Black and White Ice Cream Soda, 219
  Butter Pecan Ice Cream, 195
  Chocolate Frozen Yoghurt, 198
  Chocolate Ice Cream, 193
  Chunky Chocolate Fudge Ice Cream, 194
  Coconut Macadamia Ice Cream, 196
  Decaf-Coffee Ice Cream, 197
  Grapefruit Sorbet, 199
  Maple Walnut Ice Cream, 196
  Peach Melba Frozen Yoghurt, 197

Raspberry Rapture Ice Cream, 194
  Raspberry Sorbet, 198
  Vanilla Ice Cream, 195
Ice Lollies, 210
Irene's Turnips, 178
Italian Dressing, 99
Italian Rum Cake, 199
Ivan's Crisp Chicken, 139

Japanese Egg Custard Soup, 75–76
jellied recipes:
  Fresh Spring Salmon Mousse, 148
  Moulded Roquefort Spread, A, 81
  Strawberry-Banana Cream, 216
  Tomato Lemon Aspic, 215
Joan's Chicken Mascarpone, 135
Joan's Ricotta Sauce for Chicken, 187
Joan's Ricotta Sauce for Fish, 187
Joan's Ricotta Sauce for Pork, 187

Kayzie's Rabbit, 101
Klara's Aubergine Appetizer, 67

lamb:
  Aubergine "Little Shoes", 169–170
  Cabbage Rolls Stuffed with Meat (Dolma), 120
  Leftover Lamb or Pork Salad, 88
  Loin of Lamb with Horseradish Cream, 118
  Luscious Lamb, 117
  Moussaka, 109–110
  Stuffed Leg of Lamb, 117
Leftover Lamb or Pork Salad, 88
Lemon Barbecue Sauce, 185
Lemon-Basted Roast Chicken, 125
Lemon Chiffon Pie, 204
Lemon-Lime Mousse, 209
Lemon Sponge Cake, 201
Lime Dill Dressing, 92
liver:
  Calf's Liver in Red Wine, 110
lobster:
  Tarragon Lobster Tails, 152–153
Loin of Lamb with Horseradish Cream, 118–119
Luncheon Omelette, 54
Luscious Lamb, 117

Macadamia Nut Candy, 189

Mahoney, Nancy, M.S., R.D., iv
Manicotti, 156
Maple Walnut Ice Cream, 196
Marbled Tea Eggs, 58
Marzipan, 203
mayonnaise:
  Tomato Mayonnaise, 93
  Vinegar-Free Mayonnaise, 94
meal plans:
  for barbecues, 223
  for buffet dinners, 224
  for dessert buffets, 225
  for the Induction Diet, 20–25
  for formal dinners, 222–223
  for the Maintenance Diet, 42
  for the Ongoing Weight-Loss Diet,
    26–30
  for the Premaintenance Diet, 31–35
  for the Yeast-Free Diet, 36–41
meat recipes, 99–121
  See also bacon; beef; ham; lamb;
  liver; pepperoni; pork; rabbit; veal
metabolism, individual, 3–7
Mocha Drink, 221
Mock Potato Salad, 81–82
Moulded Roquefort Spread, 81
Most Delicious Cucumbers, The, 171
Mother's Pot Roast, 102
Moussaka, 109–110
mushrooms, regular:
  Chicken Croquettes, 130
  Gourmet Pork Chops, 112
  Honeydew and Seafood, 85
  Japanese Egg Custard Soup, 75–76
  My Grandmother's Veal Stew, 115
  Poached Fish Fillets, 142
  Porcini Mushrooms, 175
  Stuffed Courgettes with Prosciutto,
    166–167
  Veal Scallopini, 114
mushrooms, shiitake:
  Baked Scallop and Fish Soup, 77
  Chicken Cacciatore, 124
  Coq Au Vin with Shiitake
    Mushrooms, 126
  Crab and Mushroom Omelette, 55
  Cream of Shiitake Mushroom Soup,
    72–73
  Duck in Red Wine, 134
  Halibut Roll-Ups, 143

Luncheon Omelette, 54
Oriental Beef Stir Fry, 100
Oriental Chicken with Broccoli
  Rabe, 137–138
Snappy Swordfish, 141
String Beans Almandine, 163–164
Stuffed Sole, 145
Stuffed Steak, 122
Sun Luck Scallops, 140
Swede Home Fries, 177
mustard:
  Mustard Sauce, 184
  Mustard Vinaigrette, 92
  Vinegar-Free Mustard, 94
My Grandmother's Veal Stew, 115

NHANES, 2
New England Clam Chowder, 77
New England Fish Chowder, 76
Not Just Another Tossed Salad, 83
nuts:
  Almond Balls, 189
  Almond Ball Cookies, 190
  Almond Tart Pastry, 203–204
  Almond Stuffing, 133
  Butter Pecan Ice Cream, 195
  Coconut Macadamia Ice Cream,
    196
  Crab and Almond Pie, 153
  Curry Burgers, 106
  Green Beans Amandine, 167
  Macadamia Nut Candy, 189
  Maple Walnut Ice Cream, 196
  Pistachio Popcorn Balls, 190
  Toasted Nuts, 68
  Tricolour Salad with Three
    Cheeses, 91

¡Ole! Burgers, 106
Our Favourite Roquefort Dressing,
  95
Orange Cooler, 218
Oriental Beef Stir Fry, 100
Oriental Chicken with Broccoli Rabe,
  137–138
Oriental Prawns, 150

Parmesan Caesar Dressing, 99
Parsley Butter Sauce, 186
pasta recipes, 156–160

Cannelloni, 160
Enchiladas, 158
Gnocchi, 157
Green Sauce for Pasta, 183
Manicotti, 156
Pasta, 159
Pasta Sauce, 182–183
peaches:
  Peaches and Cream Omelette,
    49–50
  Peach Melba Frozen Yoghurt, 197
  Poached Peaches, 215
Peanut Butter Cookies, 211
pepperoni:
  Greek Salad, 84
pies and tarts:
  Almond Tart Pastry, 203–204
  Chocolate Mint Pie, 206
  Coconut Cream Pie, 205
  Lemon Chiffon Pie, 204
  Meringue Tart Case, 213
  Pumpkin Chiffon, 209–210
Pistachio Popcorn Balls, 190
Pizza Burgers, 104–105
Poached Fish Fillets, 142
Poached Peaches, 215
Poached Salmon Salad, 86
Porcini Mushrooms, 175
pork:
  Enchiladas, 158
  Gourmet Pork Chops, 112
  Leftover Lamb or Pork Salad, 88
  Pork Loin with Mustard, 123
  Spicy Spare Ribs, 121
  See also bacon
potato:
  Mock Potato Salad, 81–82
  Swede Home Fries, 177
poultry recipes, 124–139
Poussins:
  Gourmet Poussins, 131
prawns:
  Crunchy Seafood Salad, 90
  Honeydew and Seafood, 85
  Houston's Ceviche, 155
  Not Just Another Tossed Salad, 83
  Oriental Prawns, 150
  Prawn and Goat Cheese Omelette,
    57
  Prawns and Scallops Marc, 152

Prawns Parmesan, 151
Pumpkin Chiffon, 209–210
rabbit:
  Kayzie's Rabbit, 101
radishes:
  Crispy White Radish, 176
Raspberry Rapture Ice Cream, 194
Raspberry Sorbet, 198
Ratatouille, 173
Roast Turkey, 132
Roast Veal, 113
Rye Bread, 162

salad recipes, 79–91
  Chicken Salad, 85–86
  Chicken Salad Ham Rolls, 79
  Crunchy Seafood Salad, 90
  Coleslaw, 80
  Fresh Tuna and Avocado Salad, 80
  Greek Salad, 84
  Honeydew and Seafood, 85
  Hot Beef Salad, 87
  Leftover Lamb or Pork Salad, 88
  Mock Potato Salad, 81–82
  Moulded Roquefort Spread, 81
  Not Just Another Tossed Salad, 83
  Poached Salmon Salad, 86
  Salad Niçoise, 89–90
  Tossed Salad with Tomato
    Dressing, 82
  Tricolor Salad with Three Cheeses,
    91
salad, dressings for, 92–99
  Basic French Dressing, 95
  Basic Vinegar-Free Salad Dressing,
    93
  Creamy Celery-Seed Dressing, 97
  Curry Dressing, 98
  Dill Vinaigrette Dressing, 98
  Dressing of the House, 96
  Italian Dressing, 99
  Lime Dill Dressing, 92
  Mustard Vinaigrette, 92
  Our Favourite Roquefort Dressing,
    95
  Parmesan Caesar Dressing, 99
  Thousand Island Dressing, 97
  Tomato Mayonnaise, 93
  Vinaigrette Cream Dressing, 96
  Vinegar-Free Mayonnaise, 94

Vinegar-Free Mustard, 94
Salami and Parmesan, 62
salmon:
Fresh Spring Salmon Mousse, 148
Poached Salmon Salad, 86
Salmon Soufflé, 52
Sardine Snack, 63
sauces, 180–188
Cocktail Sauce, 181
Cheese Sauce, 186
Cranberry Sauce, 185
Cream Sauce, 180
Frozen Horseradish Cream, 180
Green Sauce for Pasta, 183
Hollandaise Sauce, 181
Hot Barbecue Sauce, 184
Joan's Ricotta Sauce for Chicken, 187
Joan's Ricotta Sauce for Fish, 187
Joan's Ricotta Sauce for Pork, 187
Lemon Barbecue Sauce, 185
Mustard Sauce, 184
Parsley Butter Sauce, 186
Pasta Sauce, 182–3
Tartare Sauce, 181
Tomato Paste, 188
Vinegar- and Sugar-Free Ketchup, 186
scallops:
Baked Scallop and Fish Soup, 77
Houston's Ceviche, 155
Prawns and Scallops Marc, 152
Sun Luck Scallops, 140
seafood. *See* fish and shellfish recipes
Shape-Up Shake, 221
shellfish. *See* fish and shellfish recipes
Snappy Swordfish, 141
sole:
Sole with Soured Cream, 144
Stuffed Sole, 145
sorbets. *See* ice cream and sorbet
soups, 69–78
Baked Scallop and Fish Soup, 77
Beef Stock, 71
Cauliflower Soup with Dill and Caraway, 78
Chicken Stock, 69
Cold Avocado Soup, 75
Cream of Chicken Soup, 70

Cream of Shiitake Mushroom Soup, 72–73
Creamy Ricotta Soup, 73
Dumplings, 72
Fish Stock, 71
Gazpacho, 74
Japanese Egg Custard Soup, 75–76
New England Clam Chowder, 77
New England Fish Chowder, 76
Vegetable Stock, 70
Soured Cream Clam Dip, 63
Spice Cake, 202
Spiced Iced Decaf Coffee, 222
Spicy Cocktail, 218
Spicy Sausage Bake, 53
Spicy Spare Ribs, 121
spinach:
Baked Spinach, 165
Not Just Another Tossed Salad, 83
Steak Au Poivre, 108
Steak Pizzaiola, 119
Strawberry-Banana Cream, 216
Stuffed Courgettes with Prosciutto, 166–167
Stuffed Leg of Lamb, 117
Stuffed Sole, 145
Stuffed Steak, 122
Stuffed Zippy Courgettes, 166
Summer Day Chicken From Spain, 128
Sun Luck Scallops, 140
swede:
Garden Beef, 116
Mock Potato Salad, 81–82
Swede Home Fries, 177
Swedish Meatballs, 60
Sweet Lemonade with Lecithin, 223
swordfish:
Snappy Swordfish, 141

Tandoori Chicken, 136
Tarragon Lobster Tails, 152–153
Tartare Sauce, 181
tarts *see* pies and tarts
Thousand Island Dressing, 97
Toasted Nuts, 68
tomatoes:
Basic Fried Green Tomatoes, 174
Cabbage Rolls Stuffed with Meat (Dolma), 120
Steak Pizzaiola, 119

Tossed Salad with Tomato Dressing, 82
Tomato Lemon Aspic, 215
Tomato Mayonnaise, 93
Tomato Purée, 188
Trout in Tomato Sauce, 147
Tossed Salad with Tomato Dressing, 82
Tricolor Salad with Three Cheeses, 91
Trout in Tomato Sauce, 147
tuna:
    Crunchy Seafood Salad, 90
    Fresh Tuna and Avocado Salad, 80
    Honeydew and Seafood, 85
    Salad Niçoise, 89–90
    Tuna Loaf, 149
turkey:
    Roast Turkey, 132
    Turkey à la King, 131–132
    Turkey Meatballs, 61
    Turkey Sausage Patties, 138
turnips:
    Irene's Turnips, 178
Two-Cheese Omelette, 55

U.S. Hamburgers, 107

Vanilla Ice Cream, 195
veal:
    My Grandmother's Veal Stew, 115
    Roast Veal, 113
    Veal Rolatine, 111
    Veal Scallopini, 114
vegetable entrées and side dishes, 164–179
    Aubergine "Little Shoes", 169–170
    Aubergine Parmigiana, 164
    Basic Fried Green Tomatoes, 174
    Baked Spinach, 165
    Broccoli with Cheese Sauce, 165
    Cauliflower Bake, 176

Cauliflower Cheese Dumplings, 168
Cheese-Stuffed Aubergine, 170
Cheesy Brussels Sprouts, 177
Chic Asparagus, 178
Chinese Mangetout, 169
Crispy White Radish, 176
Crazy Cabbage, 172
Green Beans Amandine, 167
Green Bean Chokes, 179
Irene's Turnips, 178
The Most Delicious Cucumbers, 171
Porcini Mushrooms, 175
Ratatouille, 173
Stuffed Courgettes with Prosciutto, 166–167
Stuffed Zippy Courgettes, 166
Swede Home Fries, 177
Vegetable Stock, 70
vinaigrettes
    Dill Vinaigrette Dressing, 98
    Vinaigrette Cream Dressing, 96
vinegar-free recipes:
    Basic Vinegar-Free Salad Dressing, 93
    Lime Dill Dressing, 92
    Tomato Mayonnaise, 93
    Vinegar- and Sugar-Free Ketchup, 188
    Vinegar-Free Mayonnaise, 94
    Vinegar-Free Mustard, 94

weight-loss plans:
    history of, 1–2, 18
    industry of, 2
    Weight Watchers, 2
weight regain, 4, 5

yoghurt:
    Chocolate Frozen Yoghurt, 198
    Peach Melba Frozen Yoghurt, 197